LMRVT

AF752161

PATIENT MANUAL

Lessac-Madsen Resonant Voice Therapy

Katherine Verdolini Abbott, Ph.D., CCC-SLP
Developer and author of "Lessac-Madsen Resonant Voice Therapy"

"This manual may be used as a guide for clinicians who have completed formal training in Lessac-Madsen Resonant Voice Therapy with Dr. Verdolini Abbott or a person she has designated. The material may also be used by patients, educators, and clinicians for informational and educational purposes. However, no individual may use the materials for clinical work, or claim to use the materials for clinical work, without formal training by Dr. Verdolini Abbott or a person she has designated. Such use will constitute an ethical breach and may be pursued under legal auspices."

Dedicated to Professor Arthur Lessac and Dr. Mark Madsen, whose work inspired many parts of the program and to whom I am perpetually indebted.

Plural Publishing Inc.

Contents

Lessac-Madsen Resonant Voice Therapy (LMRVT)

Note:

This manual is intended for use in voice therapy provided by a licensed speech-language pathologist trained in Lessac Madsen Resonant Voice Therapy (LMRVT) by Dr. Katherine Verdolini Abbott or another individual whom she has appointed. Clinical use of the materials by any other individual is strictly prohibited by the author.

The manual may also be used by educators and students who wish to obtain an overview of the approach and its materials. However, application of the approach or materials to clinical situations without the requisite training is prohibited.

The materials contained herein are not intended to treat or diagnose any condition.

About LMRVT

Welcome to voice therapy!

You have been referred for voice therapy because your physician found the following condition affecting your voice:

____

____

Voice therapy is often or almost always the primary treatment of choice for your condition. Your voice therapy will be provided by a licensed speech-language pathologist therapist.

____

Both experience and data tell us that you should experience improvement in your voice as a result of therapy. The amount of improvement varies from person to person, partly depending on the severity of the underlying condition, and partly depending on the patient's motivational level. We wish to assure you at the outset, however, that many patients obtain significant improvement in their voices with the general type of therapy that you will receive.

The specific type of voice therapy that you will receive is one version of a general class of therapies called "Resonant Voice Therapy." This general type of therapy is used in many clinics nationwide. Dr. Katherine Verdolini Abbott, Professor in the Department of Communication Science and Disorders and the Department of Otolaryngology at the University of Pittsburgh came to Pittsburgh from Harvard Medical School, where she developed a specific form of Resonant Voice Therapy called 'Lessac-Madsen Resonant Voice Therapy' (LMRVT). The basic premise of LMRVT is that virtually all patients who receive voice therapy or voice training have two common goals: (1) To have a strong, clear voice that can be heard over a distance and in background noise, as well as up-close; and, (2) To prevent future injury to the vocal folds, and reverse injury where it exists. Dr. Verdolini Abbott and her colleagues conducted several studies to identify a type of vocal fold biomechanics that could satisfy both of these important requirements (e.g. Berry, Verdolini Abbott, Montequin, Hess, Chan, & Titze, 2001; Verdolini, Druker, Palmer, & Samawi, 1998; Verdolini & Titze, 1995). The results indicated that when the vocal folds are barely touching or barely separated, voice should be the clearest possible, and injury should be minimized. This approach to voicing is associated with pleasant sensations, and easy, clear voice—or "resonant voice." Injury should be prevented or reversed.

> ***When the vocal folds are barely touching or barely separated, voice should be the clearest possible, and injury should be minimized.***

An initial study looking at the efficacy of resonant voice training for adults with vocal fold nodules and polyps indicates that it can, indeed, be useful in helping to improve a set of symptoms and signs associated with these conditions, which are similar to yours (Verdolini-Marston, Burke, Lessac, Glaze, & Caldwell, 1995).

Over the past few years, Dr. Verdolini Abbott developed the formal, programmatic version of "Lessac-Madsen Resonant Voice Therapy" (Verdolini Abbott, 2000) to honor two great mentors and voice teachers, Professor Arthur Lessac (1967; 1997) and Dr. Mark Madsen.

This program is modeled after a training approach shown in a recent efficacy study to optimize clinical outcomes in voice therapy for problems due to voice use (Verdolini Abbott et al., in preparation). The LMRVT program augments initial introductory approaches to "resonant voice" training to proceed to training of stronger resonant voice after a few weeks in the program. Stronger voice will involve similar pleasant sensations as for quieter resonant voice, and will feel very easy and free.

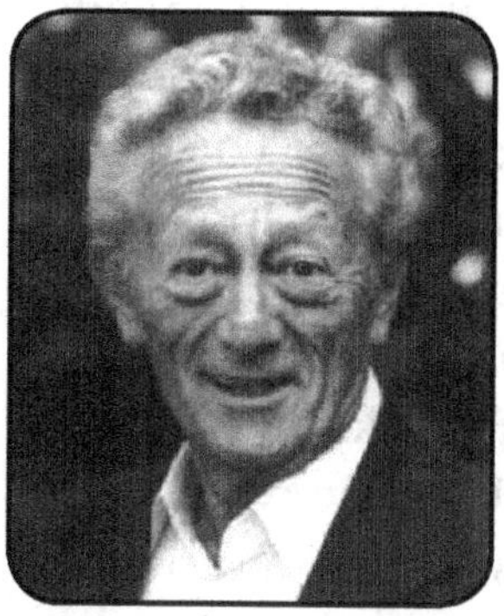

Professor Arthur Lessac

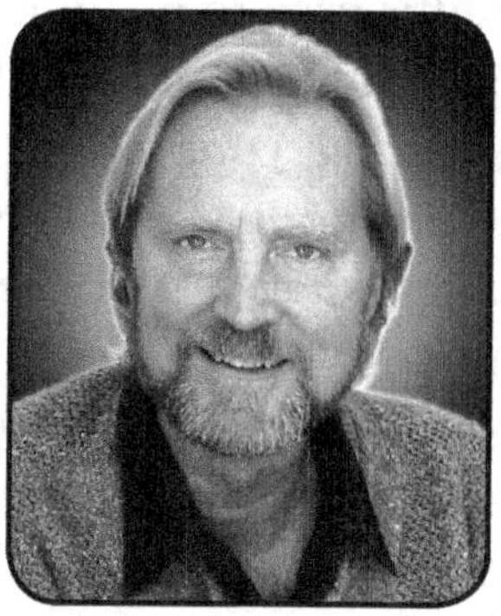

Dr. Mark Madsen

LMRVT is usually conducted during 30-45 minute sessions once or twice weekly, for 4-8 weeks. During the first therapy session, your therapist will take a few minutes to become acquainted with you and obtain information about your medical and vocal history. Together with you, your clinician will attempt to identify the specific factors that led to your particular voice problem. Then, your therapist will develop a voice care program—having to do with hydration, or reflux management, or both, that is tailor-fit to your personal needs. You will be given the program in writing in this booklet, and asked to carry it out for the duration of the therapy period or longer.

The first therapy session will end with a brief description of vocal fold vibration. The second therapy session starts with the introduction of the "Resonant Voice "Basic Training Gesture" (RV BTG). This gesture sets up the springboard for training for the remainder of therapy. You will learn how to produce voice on very simple sounds, in a way that both sounds good, and feels good. A key point in this session and throughout therapy is that your clinician will direct your attention to sensory information in voice production: What does your voice feel like? What does it sound like? The first or second therapy session will proceed with further training in the BTG, on words and phrases. Your therapist will provide you with a lot of practice on resonant voice on a large number of words and sentences, using what we call "variable practice." This type of practice should allow you to learn resonant voice very thoroughly. The result should be that you will be able to use resonant voice not only in the therapy room, but also in "real life," where it really counts, so that you can be heard with a clear and pleasant voice, and not hurt yourself while talking.

> ***Throughout therapy, your clinician will direct your attention to sensory information in voice production. What does it feel like? What does it sound like?***

The remaining therapy sessions, then, will continue to involve training in resonant voice, always emphasizing sensory processing and variable practice. About one week after completing therapy, you will receive the same voice tests that you received before therapy. We also often ask patients to come back about three months or more after you have completed therapy for final sets of tests. These tests will allow us to determine how you are doing in the long-term.

A final word about therapy regards attendance and home exercise programs. One of the most critical aspects of voice therapy success has to do with receiving therapy as it has been designed, and equally important, home practice. We can compare therapy to going to a physical trainer for overall health and fitness. In such cases, it is easy to imagine that you will obtain benefits only if you actually carry out the program that your trainer designs for you at home or in the gym. The same logic applies to voice therapy. Your therapist is essentially a "trainer," who will design a home program for you, and check it in your weekly sessions, making adjustments as needed. The work that you do between weekly therapy sessions will be the source of your greatest benefits from therapy. Of course, regular attendance is critical. Without it, therapy cannot be expected to be successful.

We look forward to working with you and helping you take charge of your vocal health: We believe that a healthier voice is just around the corner for you! LMRVT is fun and generally fruitful. Enjoy the process! Feel free to ask your therapist or your physician any questions about your care, at any time!!!

Selected References and Readings on LMRVT

Berry, D., Verdolini, K., Montequin, D., Hess, M.,Chan, R., & Titze, I.R. (2001). New indications of an optimal glottal half-width in vocal production. Journal of Speech Language and Hearing Research, 44, 29-37.

Lessac, A. (1997). The use and training of the human voice: A bio-dynamic approach to vocal life. Mountain View, CA: Mayfield Publishing.

Peterson, K.L., Verdolini-Marston, K., Barkmeier, J.M., & Hoffman, H.T. (1994). Comparison of aerodynamic and electroglottographic parameters in evaluating clinically relevant voicing patterns. Annals of Otology, Rhinology & Laryngology, 103, 335-246.

Verdolini, K. (2000). Case study: Resonant voice therapy. In Stemple, J. (2nd ed). Voice therapy: Clinical studies. pp. 46-62;82-96. Singular Publishing Group, Inc. San Diego, CA.

Verdolini, K., Druker, D.G., Palmer, P.M., & Samawi, H. (1998). Laryngeal adduction in resonant voice. Journal of Voice, 12, 315-327.

Verdolini, K., Ostrem, J., DeVore, K., McCoy, S. (1998). National Center for Voice and Speech's Guide to Vocology. NCVS. Iowa City, Iowa.

Verdolini, K., & Titze, I.R. (1995). The application of laboratory formulas to clinical voice management. American Journal of Speech Lanaguage Pathology: A Journal of Clinical Practice, 4, 62-69.

Verdolini-Marston, K., Burke, M.K., Lessac, A., Glaze, L., & Caldwell, E. (1995). A preliminary study on two methods of treatment for laryngeal nodules. Journal of Voice, 9, 74-85.

Verdolini, K., Dietrich, M., Scheffel, L., Li, N., Rosen, C.A., Branski, R.C., & Hersan, R. (in preparation). Randomized study of learning approaches in voice therapy.

Lessac-Madsen Resonant Voice Therapy (LMRVT) Protocol

Protocol

Schematic representation, prototypical LMRVT Program (30-45 minute sessions; leaving 5 min for initial "check-in" at beginning of each session and 5 min for home instructions at end of each session). See below and next pages for further information.

	Intake Hygiene (30-45 min)	Stretches (5-10 min)	RV Core (5-10 min)	RV Chant (5-10 min)	RV "VC" (5-10 min)	RV "Mini" ("VC" 5-min)	RV "Messa di voce" (5-10 min)	Converse (5-20 min)	OwnTx (15-20 min)
I	✓	(✓)	(✓)						
II		✓	✓	✓	✓			C1	
III		✓	✓	✓	✓	✓		C2	
IV		✓	✓		✓	(✓)	✓	C1+2	
V		✓	✓		✓	(✓)	✓	C3	
VI		✓	✓			(✓)	✓	C4	
VII		✓	✓				✓	C5	
VIII		✓	✓					C6	✓

C1 = normal conversation;

C2 = quiet conversation on telephone, dictaphone, or other as relevant for patient;

C3 = loud voice (over distance) as relevant for patient;

C4 = speech in background noise as relevant to patient;

C5 = emotional speech as relevant to patient;

C6 = "challenge" conversation.

Note:
This booklet is intended for use only by a Speech-Language Pathologist Trained by Dr. Verdolini Abbott in Lessac-Madsen Resonant Voice Therapy

Likely contributing factors to onset and maintenance of voice problem:

(1) ______________________________

____

(2) ______________________________

____

(3) ______________________________

____

(4) ______________________________

____

(5) ______________________________

____

Goals:

(1) Functional: ______________________________

____

(2) Medical: ______________________________

____

(3) Biomechanical : ______________________________

____

Treatment program:

Treatment type: ______________________________

How often: ______________________________

How many sessions/weeks: ______________________________

Prognosis:

____

____

Voice Care

As with most voice therapy programs, LMRVT focuses on voice production. Your therapist will first take a moment to explain the basics of voice production using visual aids. Principles of voice care are important for you in gaining and keeping vocal health. Here, review of the three most basic principles involved in Voice Care: (1) Learning how to keep the vocal fold tissue moist; (2) Learning how to keep the vocal fold tissue free from irritants; and (3) Learning to avoid frank hollering and screaming, which can really harm your vocal folds seriously, in a short period of time. Once these principles are reviewed, your clinician will develop a special "Voice Care program" that fits your specific needs.

#1 Voice Care Principle: Keeping The Vocal Folds Moist: Hydration

What is "hydration" in voice care?

In voice care, hydration involves keeping the vocal folds moist both externally and internally, and avoiding dehydration. More people are dehydrated than often realized. External dehydration may come from breathing dry air, breathing with an open mouth, smoking, and certain drying medications. In such cases, the folds can be rehydrated by inhaling steam, and possibly by using a medication called a "mucolytic" that helps to keep respiratory secretions thin and flowing. Internal dehydration comes from too much caffeine, alcohol, drying drugs, or sweating without fluid replacement. Internal rehydration is probably best achieved by drinking lots of water.

Why is hydration important for voice?

Hydration appears to affect voice in at least two ways. First, well-hydrated vocal folds vibrate with less "push" from the lungs, as compared to dry folds, especially at high pitches (e.g. Titze, 1988; Verdolini-Marston, Druker, & Titze, 1990; Verdolini, Titze, & Fennell, 1994; Verdolini et al., 2002). Second, well-hydrated vocal folds may resist injury from voice use more than dry folds, and may recover better from existing injury than dry folds (Titze, 1981; Verdolini-Marston, Sandage, & Titze, 1994).

In voice care, hydration involves keeping the vocal folds moist both externally and internally, and avoiding dehydration

Modified from Verdolini K., Ostrem J DeVore K., McCoy S., (1998). National Center for Voice and Speech's Guide to Vocology. Iowa City, Iowa: National Center for Voice and Speech.

Which types of voice conditions may benefit the most from hydration treatments, and what do the treatments consist of?

Hydration treatments may be appropriate for people with many kinds of conditions affecting voice, and are rarely harmful. However, the specific hydration program that you follow should be tailor-fit to your particular needs. For example, if your clinical examination or history indicate that you may have external vocal fold dehydration, then external rehydration (steam inhalation, use of vaporizors, etc.) may be appropriate. On the other hand, if your examination or history indicate that you are at risk for internal vocal fold dehydration, then internal—or systemic rehydration may be important for you (for example drinking lots of water. In a section that follows, your therapist will check off the types of hydration treatments that you should use. It is very important that you follow your instructions, rather than some generic "hydration" program. This is because, although rare, some hydration treatments may be harmful for some people, for medical reasons. For example, people with congestive heart failure should not drink large quantities of water without a physician's supervision, however direct steam inhalation may be alright. On the other hand, people with mold allergies can usually drink large quantities of water without any negative effects, but should not use vaporizors, because of the possibility of mold build-up in the environment. Your clinician will develop a program that is right for you.

What are my hydration instructions?

You should follow the following instructions. If a change is required at any time, your clinician will indicate this to you.

❑ Water intake daily (amount): ____________________

❑ Steam or vapor

- ❖ Shower steam (number of times daily/duriation): ____________________
- ❖ Steam inhaler (number of times daily/duration): ____________________
- ❖ Hot water vaporizor (room/daily duration): ____________________

❑ Medication (per your physician; type, dose, daily frequency): ____________________

❑ Other: ____________________

Specifics around inhaler and vaporizer use, if recommended

If your clinician recommends that you use a steam inhaler, you can purchase one at almost any drug store for $25-40. Many insurance companies will reimburse you the cost, with a physician prescription for the device. Most of the commercial devices require a small amount of water placed in a cup. Distilled water may be best by helping the device's shelf-life. You should regulate the amount of steam, and place your nose and mouth over the designated face mask. Back away from the steam if it feels to hot. Breathe in and out through your nose. A somewhat less straightforward alternative is to use a pot of water. First, boil the water on a stove or in a microwave oven. Then, remove the pot from the oven (or microwave), and place it on a table. Place your head over the pot, and surround your head with a towel. Position yourself so that the steam is not too hot. Breathe through your nose. Although less expensive than the steam device, this method does not deliver a consistent, regulated amount of steam as the device does. There is greater danger of becoming burned. Also, a steam inhaler is a handy device to have as a family health appliance in general. For example, following a physician's recommendation, it can be very useful in cases of lung or sinus congestion accompanying common colds.

If your clinician has recommended that you use a vaporizer, you should use a hot-water one, not a cool-mist device. Cool mist devices essentially vaporize everything in their reservoirs, including not only water, but also chemicals and germs. The 'white dust' that is seen on furniture and elsewhere with these devices likely ends up depositing itself on the vocal folds and in the lungs as well. In contrast, hot-water vaporizors create vapor by boiling water. Because water has a lower boiling point than most chemicals, only H_2O is delivered into the air. Most germs should be killed off. Hot-water vaporizors can be purchased at most drug stores for about $10-15. More expensive, elaborate versions which can run in the hundreds of dollars are usually not necessary. The main important warning around these vaporizors—or any vaporizor for that matter--is that they must be cleaned daily, as indicated in the manufacturer's instructions. Also, filters must be changed as indicated by the manufacturer. Otherwise, germs can build up and be dispersed in the air. If you use the device at night, you will derive the greatest benefit from a vaporizor if you turn it on about a half-hour before bedtime, and close bedroom doors and windows while it is in use. Experiment with placement relative to your bed, to find the most comfortable placement for you, which is also safe for children and pets.

If your physician indicates that you should take an over-the-counter mucolytic (a drug that thins secretions), the physician has probably cautioned you to use preparations that have only mucolytic agents (e.g. guaifenesin), without the addition of other compounds such as decongestants or antihistamines unless these are specifically prescribed. This is because such compounds have drying effects which counteract the intended moisturizing effect of the mucolytic. Commercially, Robitussin (WITHOUT INITIALS AFTER IT) is a simple mucolytic that your physician may recommend. Unless your physician specifically indicates it, you should NOT take Robitussin CM, DF, or any other "initials" as these contain the drying agents noted.

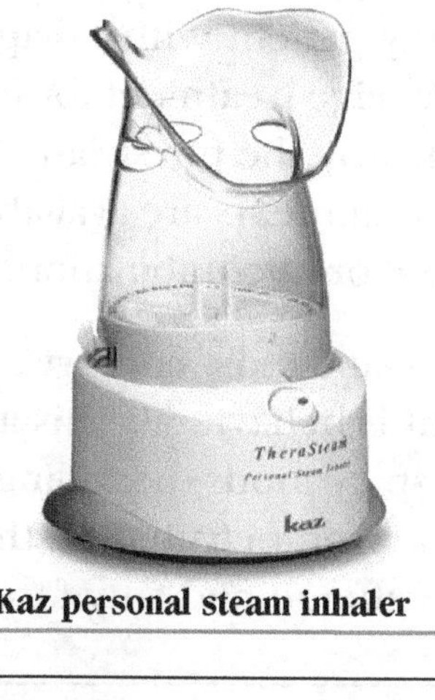

Kaz personal steam inhaler

#2 Voice Care Principle:
Keeping The Folds From Irritants: Focus on Laryngopharyngeal Reflux (LPR) and Smoking

What is LPR?

Laryngopharyngeal reflux refers to a spill-over of acids from the esophagus (food-tube) onto the vocal folds. Although the acids originally come from the stomach, LPR is somewhat different from "gastroesophageal reflux" (GER), in which stomach acids back up from the stomach into the esophagus only. Numerous studies and clinical reports have indicated that a large proportion of people with vocal pathology have LPR, which is thought to play a role in the pathology (see for example, Koufman, 1991), as discussed next.

> *Laryngopharyngeal reflux refers to a spill-over of acids from the esophagus (food-tube) onto the vocal folds.*

How does LPR affect voice?

There is wide-spread agreement that LPR can inflame the vocal folds and make people more likely to get certain vocal fold pathologies (e.g. Koufman, 1991). At the very least, LPR aggravates existing pathologies, and slows healing. There is even some speculation that LPR can affect the nerves to the vocal folds, and reduce their functioning.

Which types of voice conditions may benefit the most from LPR treatments, and what do treatments consist of?

Almost any patient with a diagnosis of LPR should receive treatment for it. The treatment is established by the physician. In general, three types of treatments are available. These may be used alone or in combination.

The first—and most conservative form of LPR treatment is behavioral. This approach involves limiting spicy foods (including tomatoes and oranges and grapefruits and their juices), alcohol, caffeine, and fatty foods (e.g. fried foods, chocolate). Patients may be instructed to sleep with their head elevated from the waist up to help keep esophageal acids from spilling into the airway during the night. The patient should not eat for at least three to four hours before lying down. If heavy around the waist, the patient should lose weight. Sometimes these precautions are enough to reduce LPR's voice symptoms.

A second form of LPR treatment involves medicines. Different types of medications can be used. One type, called H2 blockers, blocks histamine, which is one element involved in acid formation in the stomach. Examples of H2 blockers are Tagamet and Zantac. However, acid blockage is not 100% with this approach. Another class of medicines is the proton pump inhibitor. Medicines in this class block the formation of acid secretions altogether by blocking hydrogen ions, which allow stomach acid to be formed. There is typically 100% suppression of stomachacids. Examples of proton pump inhibitors are Nexium (esomeprazole magnesium), Prilosec (omeprazole) and Prevacid (lansopracole). A third class of anti-reflux drugs is the "motility drug." Medicines in this class reduce movements throughout the esophagus,

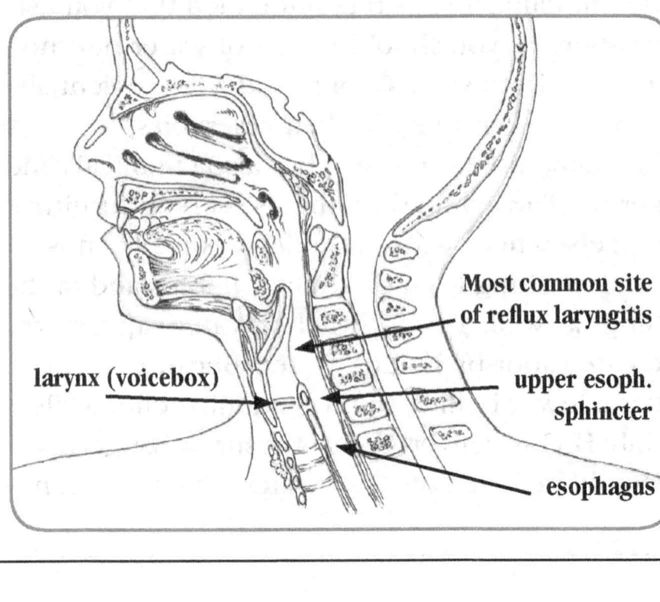

stomach, and intestines. Therefore, acids that are produced are less likely to be moved through the esophagus onto the vocal folds. Examples includes Cisipride and Propulsid. Although quite effective in the treatment of LPR, Propulsid has recently lost Federal Drug Administration approval because of its potentially serious side-effects for the heart.

A third and final form of LPR treatment is usually reserved for more persistent cases, especially those that do not get better with behavioral treatments and medicines. This approach involves very delicate surgery called "fundoplication." In this surgery, a tiny scope is inserted through the belly button. There are different methods, but basically a part of the stomach called the "fundus" is wrapped around the lower part of the esophagus, to construct a tight sphincter that keeps acids from entering the esophagus.

What are my instructions for LPR?

Your instructions have been established by your Ear-Nose-Throat physician. We re-iterate them here, at his or her instruction:

- ❑ Behavioral treatment
  - ❖ Reduce or eliminate spicy foods (including tomatoes, oranges, grapefruits), alcohol, caffeine, and fatty foods (e.g. chocolate)
  - ❖ Engage in weight reduction program
  - ❖ Do not exercise immediately after eating
  - ❖ Elevate head of bed 6
  - ❖ Do not eat for 3-4 hours before lying down
  - ❖ Do not smoke
- ❑ Drug treatment
  - ❖ Drug type:________________________
  - ❖ Drug dose:________________________
  - ❖ How often: ________________________
- ❑ Surgery: ________________________

A Few Comments About Smoking

It is probably not news to you that smoking is detrimental to your health and that smoking ranks as the most significant factor as the cause of head, neck, lung, and other cancers. On top of general health issues, smoking is also bad for your voice. Smoke is a vocal fold irritant. The chemicals in the smoke and the heat of the smoke constantly irritate the vocal fold tissues and dry them out. Over time smoke can cause long-term changes in the vocal fold mucosa. One result may be a drop in the speaking pitch or singing range. Also, various kinds of vocal fold lesions, can develop, including cancerous ones. Please also be aware of second-hand smoke. Avoid smoky environments whenever possible. Further, smoking can also increase reflux symptoms and smoking decreases lung function, which both can reduce the efficiency of the laryngeal mechanism.

You can use bricks or books, or special "wedges" purchased in health equipment stores. The use of pillows to elevate the head is not recommended, because people tend to slip off of them during the night. It is generally thought that it is important to raise the upper body during sleep, from the waist up - although there is some debate about whether this is necessary for LPR as opposed to Gastro-Esophageal Reflux, for which elevation is indeed recommended.

#3 Voice Care Principle: Screaming, Hollering, and Background Noise

What are screaming, hollering, and background noise, and how may they affect voice?

These terms are fairly self-explanatory. What is not so obvious is how often they can occur, sometimes without even knowing it. Sports events, or environments with background noise such as restaurants, bars, parties, choirs, and even church and professional gatherings may be particularly "tricky" for the voice. In these situations, you may end up using your voice much more strongly, and for much longer, than you realize. By the time the event is finished, you may discover that you are hoarse. But by that time, some damage to the vocal fold tissue may already have been done.

> *Screaming, hollering, and background noise are fairly self-explanatory. What is not so obvious is how often they can occur, sometimes without even knowing it.*

What are solutions for voice in these situations?

First of all, you should simply strike out-and-out screaming off your list of what you expect to do in your life, period. This recommendation applies not only to people with voice problems, but to everybody. The exception is clearly when danger is involved, and screaming is needed to obtain help or for defense purposes. Another exception is if you have received training in safe screaming from a specialized theatre trainer, who teaches people how to use the epiglottis (a little flap above the vocal folds) as the noise source in screaming, rather than the vocal folds. Otherwise, you should realize that every scream literally could be your last. Single, strong screams are sometimes sufficient to damage vocal fold tissue permanently, in a way that is difficult to fix later.

> *LMVRT will teach you how to use your voice strongly, so that you can speak even in background noise without hurting yourself. We emphasize, however, that you should not attempt to use your voice loudly until your clinician has specifically cleared you for it.One voice- saving "trick" is to put an ear plug in one (or two) ear(s) when you go out to be in background noise.*

Having said as much, LMRVT will teach you how to use your voice strongly, so that you can speak even in background noise without hurting yourself. We emphasize, however, that you should not attempt to use your voice loudly until your clinician has specifically cleared you for it. In the meantime, one voice-saving "trick" that you can use is to put one "swimmer's ear plug" in one ear when you go out to be in background noise. This one little plug—(a pair can be purchased at the drug store for about $2)—will increase your ability to hear your own voice in background noise. In this case, you will realize how loudly you are speaking and probably limit extreme loudnesses. In some cases you may also be able to understand what other people are saying better, as well, because the earplug may filter out some of the noise. Many, many patients have commented that this single "trick" has gone a very long way in helping them to recover from voice problems, especially people who are involved in frequent gatherings in background noise.

Selected References and Readings on Vocal Care

Fisher, K.V., Ligon, J., Sobecks, J.L., & Roxe, D.M. (2001). Phonatory effects of body fluid removal. Journal of Speech, Language and Hearing Research, 44, 354-357.

Grillo, E.U., & Verdolini, K. (in press). Evidence for distinguishing pressed, normal, resonant, and breathy voice qualities by laryngeal resistance and vocal efficiency in vocally, trained subjects. Journal of Voice.

Hemler, R.J., Wieneke, G.H., Lebacq, J., & Dejonckere, P.H. (2001). Layrngeal mucosa elasticity and viscosity in high and low relative air humidity. European Archives of Otorhinolaryngology, 258, 125-129.

Jiang, J., Verdolini, K., Acquino, B., Ng, J., & Hanson, D.G. (2000). Effects of dehydration in excised canine larynges. Annals of Otology, Rhinolgy & Laryngology, 109, 568-575.

Koufman, J.A. (1991). The otolaryngologic manifestations of gastroesophageal reflux disease (GERD): a clinical investigation of 225 patients using ambulatory 24-hour pH monitoring and an experimental investigation of the role of acid and pepsin in the development of laryngeal injury. Laryngoscope, 101(4 Pt 2 Suppl 53), 1-78.

Kjellen, G., & Brudin, L. (1994). Gastroesophageal reflux disease and laryngeal symptoms. Is there really a causal relationship? Otorhinolaryngol Relat Spec, 56, 287-290.

Lawrence, V.L. (1981). Handy household hints: To sing or not to sing. NATS Bulletin, 37, 23-25.

Sataloff, R.T. (1987). The professional voice: Part III. Common diagnoses and treatments. Journal of Voice, 1, 283-292.

Shaw, G.Y., & Searl, J.P. (1997). Laryngeal manifestations of gastroesophageal reflux before and after treatment with omeprazole. Southern Medical Journal, 90, 1115-1122.

Shaw, G.Y., Searl, J.P., Young, J.L., & Miner, P.B. (1996). Subjective, laryngoscopic, and acoustic measurements of laryngeal reflux before and after treatment with omeprazole. Journal of Voice, 10, 410-418.

Titze, I.R. (1981). Heat generation in the vocal folds and its possible effect on vocal endurance. In V.L. Lawrence (ed.), Transcripts of the Tenth Symposium: Care of the Professional Voice, Part I: Instrumentation in Voice Research (pp. 52-65). New York: The Voice Foundation.

Titze, I.R. (1988). The physics of small-amplitude oscillation of the vocal folds. Journal of the Acoustical Society of America, 83, 1536-1552.

Verdolini, K., Min, Y., Titze, I.R., Lemke, J., Brown, K., vanMersbergen, M., Fisher, K., Jiang, J. (2002). Biological mechanisms underlying voice changes due to dehydration. Journal of Speech, Language and Hearing Research, 42, 268-281.

Verdolini, K., Titze, I.R., & Fennell, A. (1994). Dependence of phonatory effort on hydration level. Journal of Speech and Hearing Research, 37, 1001-1007.

Verdolini-Marston, K., Sandage, M., & Titze, I.R. (1994). Effect of hydration treatments on laryngeal nodules and polyps and related voice measures. Journal of Voice, 8, 30-47.

Verdolini-Marston, K., Titze, I.R., & Druker, D.G. (1990). Changes in phonation threshold pressure with induced conditions of hydration. Journal of Voice, 4, 142-151.

If Sessions 1 and 2 are conducted on the same day, use the sheets for Session 1 only and omit Session 2 exercises from the home program.

SESSIONS 1-2 HOME PROGRAM **TEMPLATE**

Date: ____________________

Hydration Therapy

- ❑ Water intake daily (amount):______________________________
- ❑ Steam or vapor (indicate type/number of times daily/duration): ______________
- ❑ Medication (per your physician; type, dose, daily frequency):______________

LPR

- ❑ Behavioral treatment
  - ◆ Reduce or eliminate spicy foods, alcohol, caffeine, and fatty foods
  - ◆ Engage in weight reduction program
  - ◆ Do not exercise immediately after eating
  - ◆ Elevate head of bed 6"
  - ◆ Do not eat for 3-4 hours before lying down
  - ◆ Do not smoke
- ❑ Drug treatment (type/dose/frequency):______________________________

Stretches (2-3 min. twice daily)	RV BTG, Words, etc. (2-3 min. twice daily)	RV Chant (1-2 min. daily)	RV Messa di voce (1-2 min. daily)	RV Vocal Communicator (throughout day)	RV Minis (throughout day)
AM					
PM					

- ❑ RV BTG (Basic Training Gesture) = Sustain "mmmmm" on a comfortable pitch about 10 times.
- ❑ RV Words, Phrases, Scales = make up words starting with "mmmmm"
- ❑ RV Chant (first all on one pitch; then, repeat sentence with increasing inflection until you are on an RV "roll").
  - ◆ /Mi mi mi mi mi mi; Mi mi pi pi mi mi/; Meet me Peter, meet me
  - ◆ /Ma ma ma ma ma ma; Ma ma pa pa ma ma/; Mama, papa, mama
  - ◆ /Mu mu mu mu mu mu; Mu mu pu pu mu mu/; Mooching pooches, mooching

Do you feel vibrations? Is voice easy?

- ❑ RV Vocal Communicator = "m-hmmmmm"

Using a filled-in circle, indicate how your voice is today, overall, compared to when you first started therapy ("X" shows your rating at the start of therapy) (0 = catastrophic; 10 = exquisitely excellent).

	Start of Therapy	Today
10		
9		
8		
7		
6		
5		
4		
3		
2		
1		
0		

Other comments (successes, difficulties, etc.):______________________________

Sessions 1-2 Home Program *You Fill Out* Date: ______________

Hydration Therapy

- ❏ Water intake daily (amount): ______________
- ❏ Steam or vapor (indicate type/number of times daily/duration): ______________
- ❏ Medication (per your physician; type, dose, daily frequency): ______________

LPR

- ❏ Behavioral treatment
  - ◆ Reduce or eliminate spicy foods, alcohol, caffeine, and fatty foods
  - ◆ Engage in weight reduction program
  - ◆ Do not exercise immediately after eating
  - ◆ Elevate head of bed 6"
  - ◆ Do not eat for 3-4 hours before lying down
  - ◆ Do not smoke
- ❏ Drug treatment (type/dose/frequency): ______________

Stretches (2-3 min. twice daily)	RV BTG, Words, etc. (2-3 min. twice daily)	RV Chant (1-2 min. daily)	RV Messa di voce (1-2 min. daily)	RV Vocal Communicator (throughout day)	RV Minis (throughout day)
AM					
PM					

- ❏ RV BTG (Basic Training Gesture) = Sustain "mmmmm" on a comfortable pitch about 10 times.
- ❏ RV Words, Phrases, Scales = make up words starting with "mmmmm"
- ❏ RV Chant (first all on one pitch; then, repeat sentence with increasing inflection until you are on an RV "roll").
  - ◆ /Mi mi mi mi mi mi; Mi mi pi pi mi mi/; Meet me Peter, meet me
  - ◆ /Ma ma ma ma ma ma; Ma ma pa pa ma ma/; Mama, papa, mama
  - ◆ /Mu mu mu mu mu mu; Mu mu pu pu mu mu/; Mooching pooches, mooching
- ❏ RV Vocal Communicator = "m-hmmmmm"

Do you feel vibrations? Is voice easy?

Using a filled-in circle, indicate how your voice is today, overall, compared to when you first started therapy ("X" shows your rating at the start of therapy) (0 = catastrophic; 10 = exquisitely excellent).

	Start of Therapy	Today
10		
9		
8		
7		
6		
5		
4		
3		
2		
1		
0		

Other comments (successes, difficulties, etc.): ______________

 ____

Sessions 1-2 Home Program *You Fill Out* Date: ____________

Hydration Therapy

- ❏ Water intake daily (amount): ____________
- ❏ Steam or vapor (indicate type/number of times daily/duration): ____________
- ❏ Medication (per your physician; type, dose, daily frequency): ____________

LPR

- ❏ Behavioral treatment
  - ◆ Reduce or eliminate spicy foods, alcohol, caffeine, and fatty foods
  - ◆ Engage in weight reduction program
  - ◆ Do not exercise immediately after eating
  - ◆ Elevate head of bed 6”
  - ◆ Do not eat for 3-4 hours before lying down
  - ◆ Do not smoke
- ❏ Drug treatment (type/dose/frequency): ____________

Stretches (2-3 min. twice daily)	RV BTG, Words, etc. (2-3 min. twice daily)	RV Chant (1-2 min. daily)	RV Messa di voce (1-2 min. daily)	RV Vocal Communicator (throughout day)	RV Minis (throughout day)
AM					
PM					

- ❏ RV BTG (Basic Training Gesture) = Sustain “mmmmm” on a comfortable pitch about 10 times.
- ❏ RV Words, Phrases, Scales = make up words starting with “mmmmm”
- ❏ RV Chant (first all on one pitch; then, repeat sentence with increasing inflection until you are on an RV “roll”).
  - ◆ /Mi mi mi mi mi mi; Mi mi pi pi mi mi/; Meet me Peter, meet me
  - ◆ /Ma ma ma ma ma ma; Ma ma pa pa ma ma/; Mama, papa, mama
  - ◆ /Mu mu mu mu mu mu; Mu mu pu pu mu mu/; Mooching pooches, mooching
- ❏ RV Vocal Communicator = “m-hmmmmm”

Do you feel vibrations? Is voice easy?

Using a filled-in circle, indicate how your voice is today, overall, compared to when you first started therapy (“X” shows your rating at the start of therapy) (0 = catastrophic; 10 = exquisitely excellent).

	Start of Therapy	**Today**
10		
9		
8		
7		
6		
5		
4		
3		
2		
1		
0		

Other comments (successes, difficulties, etc.): ____________

SESSIONS 1-2 HOME PROGRAM *YOU FILL OUT* Date: ______________

Hydration Therapy

- ☐ Water intake daily (amount): ______________
- ☐ Steam or vapor (indicate type/number of times daily/duration): ______________
- ☐ Medication (per your physician; type, dose, daily frequency): ______________

LPR

- ☐ Behavioral treatment
  - ◆ Reduce or eliminate spicy foods, alcohol, caffeine, and fatty foods
  - ◆ Engage in weight reduction program
  - ◆ Do not exercise immediately after eating
  - ◆ Elevate head of bed 6"
  - ◆ Do not eat for 3-4 hours before lying down
  - ◆ Do not smoke
- ☐ Drug treatment (type/dose/frequency): ______________

Stretches (2-3 min. twice daily)	RV BTG, Words, etc. (2-3 min. twice daily)	RV Chant (1-2 min. daily)	RV Messa di voce (1-2 min. daily)	RV Vocal Communicator (throughout day)	RV Minis (throughout day)
AM					
PM					

- ☐ RV BTG (Basic Training Gesture) = Sustain "mmmmm" on a comfortable pitch about 10 times.
- ☐ RV Words, Phrases, Scales = make up words starting with "mmmmm"
- ☐ RV Chant (first all on one pitch; then, repeat sentence with increasing inflection until you are on an RV "roll").
  - ◆ /Mi mi mi mi mi mi; Mi mi pi pi mi mi/; Meet me Peter, meet me
  - ◆ /Ma ma ma ma ma ma; Ma ma pa pa ma ma/; Mama, papa, mama
  - ◆ /Mu mu mu mu mu mu; Mu mu pu pu mu mu/; Mooching pooches, mooching
- ☐ RV Vocal Communicator = "m-hmmmmm"

Do you feel vibrations? Is voice easy?

Using a filled-in circle, indicate how your voice is today, overall, compared to when you first started therapy ("X" shows your rating at the start of therapy) (0 = catastrophic; 10 = exquisitely excellent).

	Start of Therapy	Today
10		
9		
8		
7		
6		
5		
4		
3		
2		
1		
0		

Other comments (successes, difficulties, etc.): ______________

 ____

Sessions 1-2 Home Program *You Fill Out*

Date:________________

Hydration Therapy

- ❑ Water intake daily (amount):________________
- ❑ Steam or vapor (indicate type/number of times daily/duration): ________________
- ❑ Medication (per your physician; type, dose, daily frequency):________________

LPR

- ❑ Behavioral treatment
  - ◆ Reduce or eliminate spicy foods, alcohol, caffeine, and fatty foods
  - ◆ Engage in weight reduction program
  - ◆ Do not exercise immediately after eating
  - ◆ Elevate head of bed 6"
  - ◆ Do not eat for 3-4 hours before lying down
  - ◆ Do not smoke
- ❑ Drug treatment (type/dose/frequency):________________

Stretches (2-3 min. twice daily)	RV BTG, Words, etc. (2-3 min. twice daily)	RV Chant (1-2 min. daily)	RV Messa di voce (1-2 min. daily)	RV Vocal Communicator (throughout day)	RV Minis (throughout day)
AM					
PM					

- ❑ RV BTG (Basic Training Gesture) = Sustain "mmmmm" on a comfortable pitch about 10 times.
- ❑ RV Words, Phrases, Scales = make up words starting with "mmmmm"
- ❑ RV Chant (first all on one pitch; then, repeat sentence with increasing inflection until you are on an RV "roll").
  - ◆ /Mi mi mi mi mi mi; Mi mi pi pi mi mi/; Meet me Peter, meet me
  - ◆ /Ma ma ma ma ma ma; Ma ma pa pa ma ma/; Mama, papa, mama
  - ◆ /Mu mu mu mu mu mu; Mu mu pu pu mu mu/; Mooching pooches, mooching
- ❑ RV Vocal Communicator = "m-hmmmmm"

Do you feel vibrations? Is voice easy?

Using a filled-in circle, indicate how your voice is today, overall, compared to when you first started therapy ("X" shows your rating at the start of therapy) (0 = catastrophic; 10 = exquisitely excellent).

	Start of Therapy	**Today**
10		
9		
8		
7		
6		
5		
4		
3		
2		
1		
0		

Other comments (successes, difficulties, etc.):________________

SESSIONS 1-2 HOME PROGRAM ***YOU FILL OUT*** Date: ________________

Hydration Therapy

- ❑ Water intake daily (amount): ________________
- ❑ Steam or vapor (indicate type/number of times daily/duration): ________________
- ❑ Medication (per your physician; type, dose, daily frequency): ________________

LPR

- ❑ Behavioral treatment
  - ◆ Reduce or eliminate spicy foods, alcohol, caffeine, and fatty foods
  - ◆ Engage in weight reduction program
  - ◆ Do not exercise immediately after eating
  - ◆ Elevate head of bed 6"
  - ◆ Do not eat for 3-4 hours before lying down
  - ◆ Do not smoke
- ❑ Drug treatment (type/dose/frequency): ________________

Stretches (2-3 min. twice daily)	RV BTG, Words, etc. (2-3 min. twice daily)	RV Chant (1-2 min. daily)	RV Messa di voce (1-2 min. daily)	RV Vocal Communicator (throughout day)	RV Minis (throughout day)
AM					
PM					

- ❑ RV BTG (Basic Training Gesture) = Sustain "mmmmm" on a comfortable pitch about 10 times.
- ❑ RV Words, Phrases, Scales = make up words starting with "mmmmm"
- ❑ RV Chant (first all on one pitch; then, repeat sentence with increasing inflection until you are on an RV "roll").
  - ◆ /Mi mi mi mi mi mi; Mi mi pi pi mi mi/; Meet me Peter, meet me
  - ◆ /Ma ma ma ma ma ma; Ma ma pa pa ma ma/; Mama, papa, mama
  - ◆ /Mu mu mu mu mu mu; Mu mu pu pu mu mu/; Mooching pooches, mooching
- ❑ RV Vocal Communicator = "m-hmmmmm"

Do you feel vibrations?
Is voice easy?

Using a filled-in circle, indicate how your voice is today, overall, compared to when you first started therapy ("X" shows your rating at the start of therapy) (0 = catastrophic; 10 = exquisitely excellent).

	Start of Therapy	**Today**
10		
9		
8		
7		
6		
5		
4		
3		
2		
1		
0		

Other comments (successes, difficulties, etc.): ________________

Sessions 1-2 Home Program *You Fill Out* Date: ____________

Hydration Therapy

- ❑ Water intake daily (amount): ____________
- ❑ Steam or vapor (indicate type/number of times daily/duration): ____________
- ❑ Medication (per your physician; type, dose, daily frequency): ____________

LPR

- ❑ Behavioral treatment
  - ◆ Reduce or eliminate spicy foods, alcohol, caffeine, and fatty foods
  - ◆ Engage in weight reduction program
  - ◆ Do not exercise immediately after eating
  - ◆ Elevate head of bed 6"
  - ◆ Do not eat for 3-4 hours before lying down
  - ◆ Do not smoke
- ❑ Drug treatment (type/dose/frequency): ____________

Stretches (2-3 min. twice daily)	RV BTG, Words, etc. (2-3 min. twice daily)	RV Chant (1-2 min. daily)	RV Messa di voce (1-2 min. daily)	RV Vocal Communicator (throughout day)	RV Minis (throughout day)
AM					
PM					

- ❑ RV BTG (Basic Training Gesture) = Sustain "mmmmm" on a comfortable pitch about 10 times.
- ❑ RV Words, Phrases, Scales = make up words starting with "mmmmm"
- ❑ RV Chant (first all on one pitch; then, repeat sentence with increasing inflection until you are on an RV "roll").
  - ◆ /Mi mi mi mi mi mi; Mi mi pi pi mi mi/; Meet me Peter, meet me
  - ◆ /Ma ma ma ma ma ma; Ma ma pa pa ma ma/; Mama, papa, mama
  - ◆ /Mu mu mu mu mu mu; Mu mu pu pu mu mu/; Mooching pooches, mooching
- ❑ RV Vocal Communicator = "m-hmmmmm"

Do you feel vibrations? Is voice easy?

Using a filled-in circle, indicate how your voice is today, overall, compared to when you first started therapy ("X" shows your rating at the start of therapy) (0 = catastrophic; 10 = exquisitely excellent).

	Start of Therapy	Today
10		
9		
8		
7		
6		
5		
4		
3		
2		
1		
0		

Other comments (successes, difficulties, etc.): ____________

SESSIONS 1-2 HOME PROGRAM *YOU FILL OUT* Date: ____________

Hydration Therapy

- ❑ Water intake daily (amount): ____________
- ❑ Steam or vapor (indicate type/number of times daily/duration): ____________
- ❑ Medication (per your physician; type, dose, daily frequency): ____________

LPR

- ❑ Behavioral treatment
  - ◆ Reduce or eliminate spicy foods, alcohol, caffeine, and fatty foods
  - ◆ Engage in weight reduction program
  - ◆ Do not exercise immediately after eating
  - ◆ Elevate head of bed 6"
  - ◆ Do not eat for 3-4 hours before lying down
  - ◆ Do not smoke
- ❑ Drug treatment (type/dose/frequency): ____________

Stretches (2-3 min. twice daily)	RV BTG, Words, etc. (2-3 min. twice daily)	RV Chant (1-2 min. daily)	RV Messa di voce (1-2 min. daily)	RV Vocal Communicator (throughout day)	RV Minis (throughout day)
AM					
PM					

- ❑ RV BTG (Basic Training Gesture) = Sustain "mmmmm" on a comfortable pitch about 10 times.
- ❑ RV Words, Phrases, Scales = make up words starting with "mmmmm"
- ❑ RV Chant (first all on one pitch; then, repeat sentence with increasing inflection until you are on an RV "roll").
  - ◆ /Mi mi mi mi mi mi; Mi mi pi pi mi mi/; Meet me Peter, meet me
  - ◆ /Ma ma ma ma ma ma; Ma ma pa pa ma ma/; Mama, papa, mama
  - ◆ /Mu mu mu mu mu mu; Mu mu pu pu mu mu/; Mooching pooches, mooching
- ❑ RV Vocal Communicator = "m-hmmmmm"

Do you feel vibrations?
Is voice easy?

Using a filled-in circle, indicate how your voice is today, overall, compared to when you first started therapy ("X" shows your rating at the start of therapy) (0 = catastrophic; 10 = exquisitely excellent).

	Start of Therapy	Today
10		
9		
8		
7		
6		
5		
4		
3		
2		
1		
0		

Other comments (successes, difficulties, etc.): ____________

Sessions 1-2 Home Program *You Fill Out* Date: ____________

Hydration Therapy

- ❑ Water intake daily (amount): ____________
- ❑ Steam or vapor (indicate type/number of times daily/duration): ____________
- ❑ Medication (per your physician; type, dose, daily frequency): ____________

LPR

- ❑ Behavioral treatment
  - ◆ Reduce or eliminate spicy foods, alcohol, caffeine, and fatty foods
  - ◆ Engage in weight reduction program
  - ◆ Do not exercise immediately after eating
  - ◆ Elevate head of bed 6"
  - ◆ Do not eat for 3-4 hours before lying down
  - ◆ Do not smoke
- ❑ Drug treatment (type/dose/frequency): ____________

Stretches (2-3 min. twice daily)	RV BTG, Words, etc. (2-3 min. twice daily)	RV Chant (1-2 min. daily)	RV Messa di voce (1-2 min. daily)	RV Vocal Communicator (throughout day)	RV Minis (throughout day)
AM					
PM					

- ❑ RV BTG (Basic Training Gesture) = Sustain "mmmmm" on a comfortable pitch about 10 times.
- ❑ RV Words, Phrases, Scales = make up words starting with "mmmmm"
- ❑ RV Chant (first all on one pitch; then, repeat sentence with increasing inflection until you are on an RV "roll").
  - ◆ /Mi mi mi mi mi mi; Mi mi pi pi mi mi/; Meet me Peter, meet me
  - ◆ /Ma ma ma ma ma ma; Ma ma pa pa ma ma/; Mama, papa, mama
  - ◆ /Mu mu mu mu mu mu; Mu mu pu pu mu mu/; Mooching pooches, mooching
- ❑ RV Vocal Communicator = "m-hmmmmm"

Do you feel vibrations? Is voice easy?

Using a filled-in circle, indicate how your voice is today, overall, compared to when you first started therapy ("X" shows your rating at the start of therapy) (0 = catastrophic; 10 = exquisitely excellent).

	Start of Therapy	Today
10		
9		
8		
7		
6		
5		
4		
3		
2		
1		
0		

Other comments (successes, difficulties, etc.): ____________

Sessions 1-2 Home Program *You Fill Out* Date: ____________

Hydration Therapy

- ❏ Water intake daily (amount): ____________
- ❏ Steam or vapor (indicate type/number of times daily/duration): ____________
- ❏ Medication (per your physician; type, dose, daily frequency): ____________

LPR

- ❏ Behavioral treatment
  - ◆ Reduce or eliminate spicy foods, alcohol, caffeine, and fatty foods
  - ◆ Engage in weight reduction program
  - ◆ Do not exercise immediately after eating
  - ◆ Elevate head of bed 6"
  - ◆ Do not eat for 3-4 hours before lying down
  - ◆ Do not smoke
- ❏ Drug treatment (type/dose/frequency): ____________

Stretches (2-3 min. twice daily)	RV BTG, Words, etc. (2-3 min. twice daily)	RV Chant (1-2 min. daily)	RV Messa di voce (1-2 min. daily)	RV Vocal Communicator (throughout day)	RV Minis (throughout day)
AM					
PM					

- ❏ RV BTG (Basic Training Gesture) = Sustain "mmmmm" on a comfortable pitch about 10 times.
- ❏ RV Words, Phrases, Scales = make up words starting with "mmmmm"
- ❏ RV Chant (first all on one pitch; then, repeat sentence with increasing inflection until you are on an RV "roll").
  - ◆ /Mi mi mi mi mi mi; Mi mi pi pi mi mi/; Meet me Peter, meet me
  - ◆ /Ma ma ma ma ma ma; Ma ma pa pa ma ma/; Mama, papa, mama
  - ◆ /Mu mu mu mu mu mu; Mu mu pu pu mu mu/; Mooching pooches, mooching

Do you feel vibrations? Is voice easy?

- ❏ RV Vocal Communicator = "m-hmmmmm"

Using a filled-in circle, indicate how your voice is today, overall, compared to when you first started therapy ("X" shows your rating at the start of therapy) (0 = catastrophic; 10 = exquisitely excellent).

	Start of Therapy	Today
10		
9		
8		
7		
6		
5		
4		
3		
2		
1		
0		

Other comments (successes, difficulties, etc.): ____________

SESSIONS 1-2 HOME PROGRAM *YOU FILL OUT* Date: ________________

Hydration Therapy

❑ Water intake daily (amount): ____________________

❑ Steam or vapor (indicate type/number of times daily/duration): ____________________

❑ Medication (per your physician; type, dose, daily frequency): ____________________

LPR

❑ Behavioral treatment
- ◆ Reduce or eliminate spicy foods, alcohol, caffeine, and fatty foods
- ◆ Engage in weight reduction program
- ◆ Do not exercise immediately after eating
- ◆ Elevate head of bed 6"
- ◆ Do not eat for 3-4 hours before lying down
- ◆ Do not smoke

❑ Drug treatment (type/dose/frequency): ____________________

Stretches (2-3 min. twice daily)	RV BTG, Words, etc. (2-3 min. twice daily)	RV Chant (1-2 min. daily)	RV Messa di voce (1-2 min. daily)	RV Vocal Communicator (throughout day)	RV Minis (throughout day)
AM					
PM					

❑ RV BTG (Basic Training Gesture) = Sustain "mmmmm" on a comfortable pitch about 10 times.

❑ RV Words, Phrases, Scales = make up words starting with "mmmmm"

❑ RV Chant (first all on one pitch; then, repeat sentence with increasing inflection until you are on an RV "roll").

Do you feel vibrations? Is voice easy?

- ◆ /Mi mi mi mi mi mi; Mi mi pi pi mi mi/; Meet me Peter, meet me
- ◆ /Ma ma ma ma ma ma; Ma ma pa pa ma ma/; Mama, papa, mama
- ◆ /Mu mu mu mu mu mu; Mu mu pu pu mu mu/; Mooching pooches, mooching

❑ RV Vocal Communicator = "m-hmmmmm"

Using a filled-in circle, indicate how your voice is today, overall, compared to when you first started therapy ("X" shows your rating at the start of therapy) (0 = catastrophic; 10 = exquisitely excellent).

	Start of Therapy	Today
10		
9		
8		
7		
6		
5		
4		
3		
2		
1		
0		

Other comments (successes, difficulties, etc.): ____________________

____

HOME PROGRAM ***YOU FILL OUT***

Date: ____________

Hydration Therapy

❑ Water intake daily (amount): ____________

❑ Steam or vapor (indicate type/number of times daily/duration): ____________

❑ Medication (per your physician; type, dose, daily frequency): ____________

LPR

❑ Behavioral treatment
- ◆ Reduce or eliminate spicy foods, alcohol, caffeine, and fatty foods
- ◆ Engage in weight reduction program
- ◆ Do not exercise immediately after eating
- ◆ Elevate head of bed 6"
- ◆ Do not eat for 3-4 hours before lying down
- ◆ Do not smoke

❑ Drug treatment (type/dose/frequency): ____________

Stretches (2-3 min. twice daily)	RV BTG, Words, etc. (2-3 min. twice daily)	RV Chant (1-2 min. daily)	RV Messa di voce (1-2 min. daily)	RV Vocal Communicator (throughout day)	RV Minis (throughout day)
AM					
PM					

❑ RV BTG (Basic Training Gesture) = Sustain "mmmmm" on a comfortable pitch about 10 times.

❑ RV Words, Phrases, Scales = make up words starting with "mmmmm"

❑ RV Chant (first all on one pitch; then, repeat sentence with increasing inflection until you are on an RV "roll").
- ◆ /Mi mi mi mi mi mi; Mi mi pi pi mi mi/; Meet me Peter, meet me
- ◆ /Ma ma ma ma ma ma; Ma ma pa pa ma ma/; Mama, papa, mama
- ◆ /Mu mu mu mu mu mu; Mu mu pu pu mu mu/; Mooching pooches, mooching

Do you feel vibrations? Is voice easy?

❑ RV Vocal Communicator = "m-hmmmmm"

Using a filled-in circle, indicate how your voice is today, overall, compared to when you first started therapy ("X" shows your rating at the start of therapy) (0 = catastrophic; 10 = exquisitely excellent).

	Start of Therapy	Today
10		
9		
8		
7		
6		
5		
4		
3		
2		
1		
0		

Other comments (successes, difficulties, etc.): ____________

Sessions 1-2 Home Program *You Fill Out*

Date: ____________________

Hydration Therapy

- ❑ Water intake daily (amount): ____________________
- ❑ Steam or vapor (indicate type/number of times daily/duration): ____________________
- ❑ Medication (per your physician; type, dose, daily frequency): ____________________

LPR

- ❑ Behavioral treatment
  - ◆ Reduce or eliminate spicy foods, alcohol, caffeine, and fatty foods
  - ◆ Engage in weight reduction program
  - ◆ Do not exercise immediately after eating
  - ◆ Elevate head of bed 6"
  - ◆ Do not eat for 3-4 hours before lying down
  - ◆ Do not smoke
- ❑ Drug treatment (type/dose/frequency): ____________________

Stretches (2-3 min. twice daily)	RV BTG, Words, etc. (2-3 min. twice daily)	RV Chant (1-2 min. daily)	RV Messa di voce (1-2 min. daily)	RV Vocal Communicator (throughout day)	RV Minis (throughout day)
AM					
PM					

- ❑ RV BTG (Basic Training Gesture) = Sustain "mmmmm" on a comfortable pitch about 10 times.
- ❑ RV Words, Phrases, Scales = make up words starting with "mmmmm"
- ❑ RV Chant (first all on one pitch; then, repeat sentence with increasing inflection until you are on an RV "roll").
  - ◆ /Mi mi mi mi mi mi; Mi mi pi pi mi mi/; Meet me Peter, meet me
  - ◆ /Ma ma ma ma ma ma; Ma ma pa pa ma ma/; Mama, papa, mama
  - ◆ /Mu mu mu mu mu mu; Mu mu pu pu mu mu/; Mooching pooches, mooching
- ❑ RV Vocal Communicator = "m-hmmmmm"

Do you feel vibrations?
Is voice easy?

Using a filled-in circle, indicate how your voice is today, overall, compared to when you first started therapy ("X" shows your rating at the start of therapy) (0 = catastrophic; 10 = exquisitely excellent).

	Start of Therapy	Today
10		
9		
8		
7		
6		
5		
4		
3		
2		
1		
0		

Other comments (successes, difficulties, etc.): ____________________

HOME PROGRAM *YOU FILL OUT*

Date: ______________________

Hydration Therapy

- ❑ Water intake daily (amount): ______________________
- ❑ Steam or vapor (indicate type/number of times daily/duration): ______________________
- ❑ Medication (per your physician; type, dose, daily frequency): ______________________

LPR

- ❑ Behavioral treatment
  - ◆ Reduce or eliminate spicy foods, alcohol, caffeine, and fatty foods
  - ◆ Engage in weight reduction program
  - ◆ Do not exercise immediately after eating
  - ◆ Elevate head of bed 6"
  - ◆ Do not eat for 3-4 hours before lying down
  - ◆ Do not smoke
- ❑ Drug treatment (type/dose/frequency): ______________________

Stretches (2-3 min. twice daily)	RV BTG, Words, etc. (2-3 min. twice daily)	RV Chant (1-2 min. daily)	RV Messa di voce (1-2 min. daily)	RV Vocal Communicator (throughout day)	RV Minis (throughout day)
AM					
PM					

- ❑ RV BTG (Basic Training Gesture) = Sustain "mmmmm" on a comfortable pitch about 10 times.
- ❑ RV Words, Phrases, Scales = make up words starting with "mmmmm"
- ❑ RV Chant (first all on one pitch; then, repeat sentence with increasing inflection until you are on an RV "roll").
  - ◆ /Mi mi mi mi mi mi; Mi mi pi pi mi mi/; Meet me Peter, meet me
  - ◆ /Ma ma ma ma ma ma; Ma ma pa pa ma ma/; Mama, papa, mama
  - ◆ /Mu mu mu mu mu mu; Mu mu pu pu mu mu/; Mooching pooches, mooching
- ❑ RV Vocal Communicator = "m-hmmmmm"

Do you feel vibrations?
Is voice easy?

Using a filled-in circle, indicate how your voice is today, overall, compared to when you first started therapy ("X" shows your rating at the start of therapy) (0 = catastrophic; 10 = exquisitely excellent).

	Start of Therapy	**Today**
10		
9		
8		
7		
6		
5		
4		
3		
2		
1		
0		

Other comments (successes, difficulties, etc.): ______________________

Sessions 1-2 Home Program *You Fill Out*

Date: ____________________

Hydration Therapy

- ❑ Water intake daily (amount): ____________________
- ❑ Steam or vapor (indicate type/number of times daily/duration): ____________________
- ❑ Medication (per your physician; type, dose, daily frequency): ____________________

LPR

- ❑ Behavioral treatment
  - ◆ Reduce or eliminate spicy foods, alcohol, caffeine, and fatty foods
  - ◆ Engage in weight reduction program
  - ◆ Do not exercise immediately after eating
  - ◆ Elevate head of bed 6"
  - ◆ Do not eat for 3-4 hours before lying down
  - ◆ Do not smoke
- ❑ Drug treatment (type/dose/frequency): ____________________

	Stretches (2-3 min. twice daily)	RV BTG, Words, etc. (2-3 min. twice daily)	RV Chant (1-2 min. daily)	RV Messa di voce (1-2 min. daily)	RV Vocal Communicator (throughout day)	RV Minis (throughout day)
AM						
PM						

- ❑ RV BTG (Basic Training Gesture) = Sustain "mmmmm" on a comfortable pitch about 10 times.
- ❑ RV Words, Phrases, Scales = make up words starting with "mmmmm"
- ❑ RV Chant (first all on one pitch; then, repeat sentence with increasing inflection until you are on an RV "roll").
  - ◆ /Mi mi mi mi mi mi; Mi mi pi pi mi mi/; Meet me Peter, meet me
  - ◆ /Ma ma ma ma ma ma; Ma ma pa pa ma ma/; Mama, papa, mama
  - ◆ /Mu mu mu mu mu mu; Mu mu pu pu mu mu/; Mooching pooches, mooching
- ❑ RV Vocal Communicator = "m-hmmmmm"

Do you feel vibrations? Is voice easy?

Using a filled-in circle, indicate how your voice is today, overall, compared to when you first started therapy ("X" shows your rating at the start of therapy) (0 = catastrophic; 10 = exquisitely excellent).

	Start of Therapy	**Today**
10		
9		
8		
7		
6		
5		
4		
3		
2		
1		
0		

Other comments (successes, difficulties, etc.): ____________________

If Sessions 3 and 4 are conducted on the same day, use the sheets for Session 3 only and omit Session 4 exercises from the home program.

SESSIONS 3-4 HOME PROGRAM TEMPLATE

Date: ____________________

Hydration Therapy

❑ Water intake daily (amount):____________________

❑ Steam or vapor (indicate type/number of times daily/duration): ____________________

❑ Medication (per your physician; type, dose, daily frequency):____________________

LPR

❑ Behavioral treatment

- ◆ Reduce or eliminate spicy foods, alcohol, caffeine, and fatty foods
- ◆ Engage in weight reduction program
- ◆ Do not exercise immediately after eating
- ◆ Elevate head of bed 6"
- ◆ Do not eat for 3-4 hours before lying down
- ◆ Do not smoke

❑ Drug treatment (type/dose/frequency): ____________________

Stretches (2-3 min. twice daily)	RV BTG, Words, etc. (2-3 min. twice daily)	RV Chant (1-2 min. daily)	RV Messa di voce (1-2 min. daily)	RV Vocal Communicator (throughout day)	RV Minis (throughout day)
AM					
PM					

❑ RV BTG (Basic Training Gesture) = Sustain "mmmmm" on a comfortable pitch about 10 times.

❑ RV Words, Phrases, Scales = make up words starting with "nnnn";"gegegege";"rrrrr";"llllll"; "zzzzz";"vvvvv"; ngngngng";"mmmm"

❑ RV Chant (first all on one pitch; then, repeat sentence with increasing inflection until you are on an RV "roll").: No no no no no no; no no to to no no; no no, Toto, no no! /zi zi zi zi zi zi; zi zi si si zi zi/; Ziti Sissy, ziti! /vu vu vu vu vu vu; vu vu fu fu vu vu/; Voodoo, foolish voodoo!

Do you feel vibrations? Is voice easy?

❑ RV Vocal Communicator = "m-hmmm", "really", "right", "yeah", "no"

❑ RV Mini. "pull out" to RV; at phrase or other boundary, switch positions, take a breath, and come back in with strong RV:

Using a filled-in circle, indicate how your voice is today, overall, compared to when you first started therapy ("X" shows your rating at the start of therapy) (0 = catastrophic; 10 = exquisitely excellent).

	Start of Therapy	Today
10		
9		
8		
7		
6		
5		
4		
3		
2		
1		
0		

Other comments (successes, difficulties, etc.):____________________

SESSIONS 3-4 HOME PROGRAM *YOU FILL OUT* Date:____________

Hydration Therapy

- ❑ Water intake daily (amount):____________
- ❑ Steam or vapor (indicate type/number of times daily/duration): ____________
- ❑ Medication (per your physician; type, dose, daily frequency): ____________

LPR

❑ Behavioral treatment
- ◆ Reduce or eliminate spicy foods, alcohol, caffeine, and fatty foods
- ◆ Engage in weight reduction program
- ◆ Do not exercise immediately after eating
- ◆ Elevate head of bed 6"
- ◆ Do not eat for 3-4 hours before lying down
- ◆ Do not smoke

❑ Drug treatment (type/dose/frequency): ____________

Stretches (2-3 min. twice daily)	RV BTG, Words, etc. (2-3 min. twice daily)	RV Chant (1-2 min. daily)	RV Messa di voce (1-2 min. daily)	RV Vocal Communicator (throughout day)	RV Minis (throughout day)
AM					
PM					

- ❑ RV BTG (Basic Training Gesture) = Sustain "mmmmm" on a comfortable pitch about 10 times.
- ❑ RV Words, Phrases, Scales = make up words starting with "nnnn";"gegegege";"rrrrr";"llllll"; "zzzzz";"vvvvv"; ngngngng";"mmmm"
- ❑ RV Chant (first all on one pitch; then, repeat sentence with increasing inflection until you are on an RV "roll").: No no no no no no; no no to to no no; no no, Toto, no no! /zi zi zi zi zi zi; zi zi si si zi zi/; Ziti Sissy, ziti! /vu vu vu vu vu vu; vu vu fu fu vu vu/; Voodoo, foolish voodoo!
- ❑ RV Vocal Communicator = "m-hmmm", "really", "right", "yeah", "no"
- ❑ RV Mini. "pull out" to RV; at phrase or other boundary, switch positions, take a breath, and come back in with strong RV:

Do you feel vibrations? Is voice easy?

Using a filled-in circle, indicate how your voice is today, overall, compared to when you first started therapy ("X" shows your rating at the start of therapy) (0 = catastrophic; 10 = exquisitely excellent).

	Start of Therapy	**Today**
10		
9		
8		
7		
6		
5		
4		
3		
2		
1		
0		

Other comments (successes, difficulties, etc.): ____________

Sessions 3-4 Home Program *You Fill Out* Date:________________

Hydration Therapy

- ❑ Water intake daily (amount):________________
- ❑ Steam or vapor (indicate type/number of times daily/duration): ________________
- ❑ Medication (per your physician; type, dose, daily frequency):________________

LPR

- ❑ Behavioral treatment
  - ◆ Reduce or eliminate spicy foods, alcohol, caffeine, and fatty foods
  - ◆ Engage in weight reduction program
  - ◆ Do not exercise immediately after eating
  - ◆ Elevate head of bed 6"
  - ◆ Do not eat for 3-4 hours before lying down
  - ◆ Do not smoke
- ❑ Drug treatment (type/dose/frequency): ________________

Stretches (2-3 min. twice daily)	RV BTG, Words, etc. (2-3 min. twice daily)	RV Chant (1-2 min. daily)	RV Messa di voce (1-2 min. daily)	RV Vocal Communicator (throughout day)	RV Minis (throughout day)
AM					
PM					

- ❑ RV BTG (Basic Training Gesture) = Sustain "mmmmm" on a comfortable pitch about 10 times.
- ❑ RV Words, Phrases, Scales = make up words starting with "nnnn";"gegegege";"rrrrr";"llllll"; "zzzzz";"vvvvv"; ngngngng";"mmmm"
- ❑ RV Chant (first all on one pitch; then, repeat sentence with increasing inflection until you are on an RV "roll").: No no no no no no; no no to to no no; no no, Toto, no no! /zi zi zi zi zi zi; zi zi si si zi zi/; Ziti Sissy, ziti! /vu vu vu vu vu vu; vu vu fu fu vu vu/; Voodoo, foolish voodoo!
- ❑ RV Vocal Communicator = "m-hmmm","really","right","yeah","no"
- ❑ RV Mini."pull out" to RV; at phrase or other boundary, switch positions, take a breath, and come back in with strong RV:

Do you feel vibrations? Is voice easy?

Using a filled-in circle, indicate how your voice is today, overall, compared to when you first started therapy ("X" shows your rating at the start of therapy) (0 = catastrophic; 10 = exquisitely excellent).

	Start of Therapy	**Today**
10		
9		
8		
7		
6		
5		
4		
3		
2		
1		
0		

Other comments (successes, difficulties, etc.):________________

Sessions 3-4 Home Program *You Fill Out* Date:___________

Hydration Therapy

- ❑ Water intake daily (amount):___________
- ❑ Steam or vapor (indicate type/number of times daily/duration): ___________
- ❑ Medication (per your physician; type, dose, daily frequency): ___________

LPR

- ❑ Behavioral treatment
  - ◆ Reduce or eliminate spicy foods, alcohol, caffeine, and fatty foods
  - ◆ Engage in weight reduction program
  - ◆ Do not exercise immediately after eating
  - ◆ Elevate head of bed 6"
  - ◆ Do not eat for 3-4 hours before lying down
  - ◆ Do not smoke
- ❑ Drug treatment (type/dose/frequency): ___________

Stretches (2-3 min. twice daily)	RV BTG, Words, etc. (2-3 min. twice daily)	RV Chant (1-2 min. daily)	RV Messa di voce (1-2 min. daily)	RV Vocal Communicator (throughout day)	RV Minis (throughout day)
AM					
PM					

- ❑ RV BTG (Basic Training Gesture) = Sustain "mmmmm" on a comfortable pitch about 10 times.
- ❑ RV Words, Phrases, Scales = make up words starting with "nnnn";"gegegege";"rrrrr";"llllll"; "zzzzz";"vvvvv"; ngngngng";"mmmm"
- ❑ RV Chant (first all on one pitch; then, repeat sentence with increasing inflection until you are on an RV "roll").: No no no no no no; no no to to no no; no no, Toto, no no! /zi zi zi zi zi zi; zi zi si si zi zi/; Ziti Sissy, ziti! /vu vu vu vu vu vu; vu vu fu fu vu vu/; Voodoo, foolish voodoo!
- ❑ RV Vocal Communicator = "m-hmmm", "really", "right", "yeah", "no"
- ❑ RV Mini. "pull out" to RV; at phrase or other boundary, switch positions, take a breath, and come back in with strong RV:

Do you feel vibrations? Is voice easy?

Using a filled-in circle, indicate how your voice is today, overall, compared to when you first started therapy ("X" shows your rating at the start of therapy) (0 = catastrophic; 10 = exquisitely excellent).

	Start of Therapy	**Today**
10		
9		
8		
7		
6		
5		
4		
3		
2		
1		
0		

Other comments (successes, difficulties, etc.): ___________

Sessions 3-4 Home Program *You Fill Out*

Date:____________________

Hydration Therapy

❑ Water intake daily (amount):______________________________

❑ Steam or vapor (indicate type/number of times daily/duration): ______________

❑ Medication (per your physician; type, dose, daily frequency):______________

LPR

❑ Behavioral treatment

- Reduce or eliminate spicy foods, alcohol, caffeine, and fatty foods
- Engage in weight reduction program
- Do not exercise immediately after eating
- Elevate head of bed 6"
- Do not eat for 3-4 hours before lying down
- Do not smoke

❑ Drug treatment (type/dose/frequency):______________________________

Stretches (2-3 min. twice daily)	RV BTG, Words, etc. (2-3 min. twice daily)	RV Chant (1-2 min. daily)	RV Messa di voce (1-2 min. daily)	RV Vocal Communicator (throughout day)	RV Minis (throughout day)
AM					
PM					

❑ RV BTG (Basic Training Gesture) = Sustain "mmmmm" on a comfortable pitch about 10 times.

❑ RV Words, Phrases, Scales = make up words starting with "nnnn";"gegegege";"rrrrr";"lllll"; "zzzzz";"vvvvv"; ngngngng";"mmmm"

❑ RV Chant (first all on one pitch; then, repeat sentence with increasing inflection until you are on an RV "roll").: No no no no no no; no no to to no no; no no, Toto, no no! /zi zi zi zi zi zi; zi zi si si zi zi/; Ziti Sissy, ziti! /vu vu vu vu vu vu; vu vu fu fu vu vu/; Voodoo, foolish voodoo!

❑ RV Vocal Communicator = "m-hmmm", "really", "right", "yeah", "no"

Do you feel vibrations? Is voice easy?

❑ RV Mini. "pull out" to RV; at phrase or other boundary, switch positions, take a breath, and come back in with strong RV:

Using a filled-in circle, indicate how your voice is today, overall, compared to when you first started therapy ("X" shows your rating at the start of therapy) (0 = catastrophic; 10 = exquisitely excellent).

	Start of Therapy	Today
10		
9		
8		
7		
6		
5		
4		
3		
2		
1		
0		

Other comments (successes, difficulties, etc.):______________________________

 Date:________________

Hydration Therapy

❑ Water intake daily (amount):________________

❑ Steam or vapor (indicate type/number of times daily/duration): ________________

❑ Medication (per your physician; type, dose, daily frequency): ________________

LPR

❑ Behavioral treatment
- ◆ Reduce or eliminate spicy foods, alcohol, caffeine, and fatty foods
- ◆ Engage in weight reduction program
- ◆ Do not exercise immediately after eating
- ◆ Elevate head of bed 6"
- ◆ Do not eat for 3-4 hours before lying down
- ◆ Do not smoke

❑ Drug treatment (type/dose/frequency): ________________

Stretches (2-3 min. twice daily)	RV BTG, Words, etc. (2-3 min. twice daily)	RV Chant (1-2 min. daily)	RV Messa di voce (1-2 min. daily)	RV Vocal Communicator (throughout day)	RV Minis (throughout day)
AM					
PM					

❑ RV BTG (Basic Training Gesture) = Sustain "mmmmm" on a comfortable pitch about 10 times.

❑ RV Words, Phrases, Scales = make up words starting with "nnnn";"gegegege";"rrrrr";"llllll"; "zzzzz";"vvvvv"; ngngngng";"mmmm"

❑ RV Chant (first all on one pitch; then, repeat sentence with increasing inflection until you are on an RV "roll").: No no no no no no; no no to to no no; no no, Toto, no no! /zi zi zi zi zi zi; zi zi si si zi zi/; Ziti Sissy, ziti! /vu vu vu vu vu vu; vu vu fu fu vu vu/; Voodoo, foolish voodoo!

❑ RV Vocal Communicator = "m-hmmm", "really", "right", "yeah", "no"

Do you feel vibrations? Is voice easy?

❑ RV Mini. "pull out" to RV; at phrase or other boundary, switch positions, take a breath, and come back in with strong RV:

Using a filled-in circle, indicate how your voice is today, overall, compared to when you first started therapy ("X" shows your rating at the start of therapy) (0 = catastrophic; 10 = exquisitely excellent).

	Start of Therapy	**Today**
10		
9		
8		
7		
6		
5		
4		
3		
2		
1		
0		

Other comments (successes, difficulties, etc.): ________________

Sessions 3-4 Home Program *You Fill Out* Date:____________

Hydration Therapy

❑ Water intake daily (amount):____________

❑ Steam or vapor (indicate type/number of times daily/duration): ____________

❑ Medication (per your physician; type, dose, daily frequency):____________

LPR

❑ Behavioral treatment

- Reduce or eliminate spicy foods, alcohol, caffeine, and fatty foods
- Engage in weight reduction program
- Do not exercise immediately after eating
- Elevate head of bed 6"
- Do not eat for 3-4 hours before lying down
- Do not smoke

❑ Drug treatment (type/dose/frequency):____________

Stretches (2-3 min. twice daily)	RV BTG, Words, etc. (2-3 min. twice daily)	RV Chant (1-2 min. daily)	RV Messa di voce (1-2 min. daily)	RV Vocal Communicator (throughout day)	RV Minis (throughout day)
AM					
PM					

❑ RV BTG (Basic Training Gesture) = Sustain "mmmmm" on a comfortable pitch about 10 times.

❑ RV Words, Phrases, Scales = make up words starting with "nnnn";"gegegege";"rrrrr";"lllll"; "zzzzz";"vvvvv"; ngngngng";"mmmm"

❑ RV Chant (first all on one pitch; then, repeat sentence with increasing inflection until you are on an RV "roll").: No no no no no no; no no to to no no; no no, Toto, no no! /zi zi zi zi zi zi; zi zi si si zi zi/; Ziti Sissy, ziti! /vu vu vu vu vu vu; vu vu fu fu vu vu/; Voodoo, foolish voodoo!

❑ RV Vocal Communicator = "m-hmmm", "really", "right", "yeah", "no"

Do you feel vibrations? Is voice easy?

❑ RV Mini. "pull out" to RV; at phrase or other boundary, switch positions, take a breath, and come back in with strong RV:

Using a filled-in circle, indicate how your voice is today, overall, compared to when you first started therapy ("X" shows your rating at the start of therapy) (0 = catastrophic; 10 = exquisitely excellent).

	Start of Therapy	**Today**
10		
9		
8		
7		
6		
5		
4		
3		
2		
1		
0		

Other comments (successes, difficulties, etc.):____________

SESSIONS 3-4 HOME PROGRAM *YOU FILL OUT* Date:___________

Hydration Therapy

- ❑ Water intake daily (amount):___________
- ❑ Steam or vapor (indicate type/number of times daily/duration): ___________
- ❑ Medication (per your physician; type, dose, daily frequency): ___________

LPR

- ❑ Behavioral treatment
  - ◆ Reduce or eliminate spicy foods, alcohol, caffeine, and fatty foods
  - ◆ Engage in weight reduction program
  - ◆ Do not exercise immediately after eating
  - ◆ Elevate head of bed 6"
  - ◆ Do not eat for 3-4 hours before lying down
  - ◆ Do not smoke
- ❑ Drug treatment (type/dose/frequency): ___________

Stretches (2-3 min. twice daily)	RV BTG, Words, etc. (2-3 min. twice daily)	RV Chant (1-2 min. daily)	RV Messa di voce (1-2 min. daily)	RV Vocal Communicator (throughout day)	RV Minis (throughout day)
AM					
PM					

- ❑ RV BTG (Basic Training Gesture) = Sustain "mmmmm" on a comfortable pitch about 10 times.
- ❑ RV Words, Phrases, Scales = make up words starting with "nnnn";"gegegege";"rrrrr";"llllll"; "zzzzz";"vvvvv"; ngngngng";"mmmm"
- ❑ RV Chant (first all on one pitch; then, repeat sentence with increasing inflection until you are on an RV "roll").: No no no no no no; no no to to no no; no no, Toto, no no! /zi zi zi zi zi zi; zi zi si si zi zi/; Ziti Sissy, ziti! /vu vu vu vu vu vu; vu vu fu fu vu vu/; Voodoo, foolish voodoo!
- ❑ RV Vocal Communicator = "m-hmmm", "really", "right", "yeah", "no"
- ❑ RV Mini. "pull out" to RV; at phrase or other boundary, switch positions, take a breath, and come back in with strong RV:

Do you feel vibrations? Is voice easy?

Using a filled-in circle, indicate how your voice is today, overall, compared to when you first started therapy ("X" shows your rating at the start of therapy) (0 = catastrophic; 10 = exquisitely excellent).

	Start of Therapy	**Today**
10		
9		
8		
7		
6		
5		
4		
3		
2		
1		
0		

Other comments (successes, difficulties, etc.): ___________

SESSIONS 3-4 HOME PROGRAM *YOU FILL OUT*

Date:______________

Hydration Therapy

- ❑ Water intake daily (amount):______________
- ❑ Steam or vapor (indicate type/number of times daily/duration): ______________
- ❑ Medication (per your physician; type, dose, daily frequency):______________

LPR

- ❑ Behavioral treatment
  - ◆ Reduce or eliminate spicy foods, alcohol, caffeine, and fatty foods
  - ◆ Engage in weight reduction program
  - ◆ Do not exercise immediately after eating
  - ◆ Elevate head of bed 6"
  - ◆ Do not eat for 3-4 hours before lying down
  - ◆ Do not smoke
- ❑ Drug treatment (type/dose/frequency):______________

Stretches (2-3 min. twice daily)	RV BTG, Words, etc. (2-3 min. twice daily)	RV Chant (1-2 min. daily)	RV Messa di voce (1-2 min. daily)	RV Vocal Communicator (throughout day)	RV Minis (throughout day)
AM					
PM					

- ❑ RV BTG (Basic Training Gesture) = Sustain "mmmmm" on a comfortable pitch about 10 times.
- ❑ RV Words, Phrases, Scales = make up words starting with "nnnn";"gegegege";"rrrrr";"llllll"; "zzzzz";"vvvvv"; ngngngng";"mmmm"
- ❑ RV Chant (first all on one pitch; then, repeat sentence with increasing inflection until you are on an RV "roll").: No no no no no no; no no to to no no; no no, Toto, no no! /zi zi zi zi zi zi; zi zi si si zi zi/; Ziti Sissy, ziti! /vu vu vu vu vu vu; vu vu fu fu vu vu/; Voodoo, foolish voodoo!
- ❑ RV Vocal Communicator = "m-hmmm", "really", "right", "yeah", "no"
- ❑ RV Mini. "pull out" to RV; at phrase or other boundary, switch positions, take a breath, and come back in with strong RV:

Do you feel vibrations? Is voice easy?

Using a filled-in circle, indicate how your voice is today, overall, compared to when you first started therapy ("X" shows your rating at the start of therapy) (0 = catastrophic; 10 = exquisitely excellent).

	Start of Therapy	Today
10		
9		
8		
7		
6		
5		
4		
3		
2		
1		
0		

Other comments (successes, difficulties, etc.):______________

SESSIONS 3-4 HOME PROGRAM *YOU FILL OUT* Date:____________

Hydration Therapy

- ❑ Water intake daily (amount):____________
- ❑ Steam or vapor (indicate type/number of times daily/duration): ____________
- ❑ Medication (per your physician; type, dose, daily frequency): ____________

LPR

- ❑ Behavioral treatment
  - ◆ Reduce or eliminate spicy foods, alcohol, caffeine, and fatty foods
  - ◆ Engage in weight reduction program
  - ◆ Do not exercise immediately after eating
  - ◆ Elevate head of bed 6”
  - ◆ Do not eat for 3-4 hours before lying down
  - ◆ Do not smoke
- ❑ Drug treatment (type/dose/frequency): ____________

Stretches (2-3 min. twice daily)	RV BTG, Words, etc. (2-3 min. twice daily)	RV Chant (1-2 min. daily)	RV Messa di voce (1-2 min. daily)	RV Vocal Communicator (throughout day)	RV Minis (throughout day)
AM					
PM					

- ❑ RV BTG (Basic Training Gesture) = Sustain “mmmmm” on a comfortable pitch about 10 times.
- ❑ RV Words, Phrases, Scales = make up words starting with “nnnn”; “gegegege”; “rrrrr”; “lllll”; “zzzzz”; “vvvvv”; ngngngng”; “mmmm”
- ❑ RV Chant (first all on one pitch; then, repeat sentence with increasing inflection until you are on an RV “roll”).: No no no no no no; no no to to no no; no no, Toto, no no! /zi zi zi zi zi zi; zi zi si si zi zi/; Ziti Sissy, ziti! /vu vu vu vu vu vu; vu vu fu fu vu vu/; Voodoo, foolish voodoo!
- ❑ RV Vocal Communicator = “m-hmmm”, “really”, “right”, “yeah”, “no”
- ❑ RV Mini. “pull out” to RV; at phrase or other boundary, switch positions, take a breath, and come back in with strong RV:

Do you feel vibrations? Is voice easy?

Using a filled-in circle, indicate how your voice is today, overall, compared to when you first started therapy (“X” shows your rating at the start of therapy) (0 = catastrophic; 10 = exquisitely excellent).

	Start of Therapy	**Today**
10		
9		
8		
7		
6		
5		
4		
3		
2		
1		
0		

Other comments (successes, difficulties, etc.): ____________

Sessions 3-4 Home Program *You Fill Out* Date:____________

Hydration Therapy

- ❑ Water intake daily (amount):____________
- ❑ Steam or vapor (indicate type/number of times daily/duration): ____________
- ❑ Medication (per your physician; type, dose, daily frequency):____________

LPR

- ❑ Behavioral treatment
  - ◆ Reduce or eliminate spicy foods, alcohol, caffeine, and fatty foods
  - ◆ Engage in weight reduction program
  - ◆ Do not exercise immediately after eating
  - ◆ Elevate head of bed 6"
  - ◆ Do not eat for 3-4 hours before lying down
  - ◆ Do not smoke
- ❑ Drug treatment (type/dose/frequency):____________

Stretches (2-3 min. twice daily)	RV BTG, Words, etc. (2-3 min. twice daily)	RV Chant (1-2 min. daily)	RV Messa di voce (1-2 min. daily)	RV Vocal Communicator (throughout day)	RV Minis (throughout day)
AM					
PM					

- ❑ RV BTG (Basic Training Gesture) = Sustain "mmmmm" on a comfortable pitch about 10 times.
- ❑ RV Words, Phrases, Scales = make up words starting with "nnnn";"gegegege";"rrrrr";"llllll"; "zzzzz";"vvvvv"; ngngngng";"mmmm"
- ❑ RV Chant (first all on one pitch; then, repeat sentence with increasing inflection until you are on an RV "roll").: No no no no no no; no no to to no no; no no, Toto, no no! /zi zi zi zi zi zi; zi zi si si zi zi/; Ziti Sissy, ziti! /vu vu vu vu vu vu; vu vu fu fu vu vu/; Voodoo, foolish voodoo!
- ❑ RV Vocal Communicator = "m-hmmm","really","right","yeah","no"
- ❑ RV Mini."pull out" to RV; at phrase or other boundary, switch positions, take a breath, and come back in with strong RV:

Do you feel vibrations? Is voice easy?

Using a filled-in circle, indicate how your voice is today, overall, compared to when you first started therapy ("X" shows your rating at the start of therapy) (0 = catastrophic; 10 = exquisitely excellent).

	Start of Therapy	**Today**
10		
9		
8		
7		
6		
5		
4		
3		
2		
1		
0		

Other comments (successes, difficulties, etc.):____________

SESSIONS 3-4 HOME PROGRAM *YOU FILL OUT* Date:________________

Hydration Therapy

❑ Water intake daily (amount):________________

❑ Steam or vapor (indicate type/number of times daily/duration): ________________

❑ Medication (per your physician; type, dose, daily frequency):________________

LPR

❑ Behavioral treatment
- ◆ Reduce or eliminate spicy foods, alcohol, caffeine, and fatty foods
- ◆ Engage in weight reduction program
- ◆ Do not exercise immediately after eating
- ◆ Elevate head of bed 6"
- ◆ Do not eat for 3-4 hours before lying down
- ◆ Do not smoke

❑ Drug treatment (type/dose/frequency): ________________

Stretches (2-3 min. twice daily)	RV BTG, Words, etc. (2-3 min. twice daily)	RV Chant (1-2 min. daily)	RV Messa di voce (1-2 min. daily)	RV Vocal Communicator (throughout day)	RV Minis (throughout day)
AM					
PM					

❑ RV BTG (Basic Training Gesture) = Sustain "mmmmm" on a comfortable pitch about 10 times.

❑ RV Words, Phrases, Scales = make up words starting with "nnnn";"gegegege";"rrrrr";"lllll"; "zzzzz";"vvvvv"; ngngngng";"mmmm"

❑ RV Chant (first all on one pitch; then, repeat sentence with increasing inflection until you are on an RV "roll").: No no no no no no; no no to to no no; no no, Toto, no no! /zi zi zi zi zi zi; zi zi si si zi zi/; Ziti Sissy, ziti! /vu vu vu vu vu vu; vu vu fu fu vu vu/; Voodoo, foolish voodoo!

❑ RV Vocal Communicator = "m-hmmm", "really", "right", "yeah", "no"

Do you feel vibrations? Is voice easy?

❑ RV Mini. "pull out" to RV; at phrase or other boundary, switch positions, take a breath, and come back in with strong RV:

Using a filled-in circle, indicate how your voice is today, overall, compared to when you first started therapy ("X" shows your rating at the start of therapy) (0 = catastrophic; 10 = exquisitely excellent).

	Start of Therapy	Today
10		
9		
8		
7		
6		
5		
4		
3		
2		
1		
0		

Other comments (successes, difficulties, etc.): ________________

____

Sessions 3-4 Home Program *You Fill Out* Date:____________

Hydration Therapy

- ❑ Water intake daily (amount):____________
- ❑ Steam or vapor (indicate type/number of times daily/duration): ____________
- ❑ Medication (per your physician; type, dose, daily frequency):____________

LPR

- ❑ Behavioral treatment
  - ◆ Reduce or eliminate spicy foods, alcohol, caffeine, and fatty foods
  - ◆ Engage in weight reduction program
  - ◆ Do not exercise immediately after eating
  - ◆ Elevate head of bed 6"
  - ◆ Do not eat for 3-4 hours before lying down
  - ◆ Do not smoke
- ❑ Drug treatment (type/dose/frequency):____________

Stretches (2-3 min. twice daily)	RV BTG, Words, etc. (2-3 min. twice daily)	RV Chant (1-2 min. daily)	RV Messa di voce (1-2 min. daily)	RV Vocal Communicator (throughout day)	RV Minis (throughout day)
AM					
PM					

- ❑ RV BTG (Basic Training Gesture) = Sustain "mmmmm" on a comfortable pitch about 10 times.
- ❑ RV Words, Phrases, Scales = make up words starting with "nnnn";"gegegege";"rrrrr";"llllll"; "zzzzz";"vvvvv"; ngngngng";"mmmm"
- ❑ RV Chant (first all on one pitch; then, repeat sentence with increasing inflection until you are on an RV "roll").: No no no no no no; no no to to no no; no no, Toto, no no! /zi zi zi zi zi zi; zi zi si si zi zi/; Ziti Sissy, ziti! /vu vu vu vu vu vu; vu vu fu fu vu vu/; Voodoo, foolish voodoo!
- ❑ RV Vocal Communicator = "m-hmmm", "really", "right", "yeah", "no"
- ❑ RV Mini. "pull out" to RV; at phrase or other boundary, switch positions, take a breath, and come back in with strong RV:

Do you feel vibrations? Is voice easy?

Using a filled-in circle, indicate how your voice is today, overall, compared to when you first started therapy ("X" shows your rating at the start of therapy) (0 = catastrophic; 10 = exquisitely excellent).

	Start of Therapy	Today
10		
9		
8		
7		
6		
5		
4		
3		
2		
1		
0		

Other comments (successes, difficulties, etc.):____________

Sessions 3-4 Home Program *You Fill Out* Date:____________

Hydration Therapy

❑ Water intake daily (amount):____________

❑ Steam or vapor (indicate type/number of times daily/duration): ____________

❑ Medication (per your physician; type, dose, daily frequency):____________

LPR

❑ Behavioral treatment
- ◆ Reduce or eliminate spicy foods, alcohol, caffeine, and fatty foods
- ◆ Engage in weight reduction program
- ◆ Do not exercise immediately after eating
- ◆ Elevate head of bed 6"
- ◆ Do not eat for 3-4 hours before lying down
- ◆ Do not smoke

❑ Drug treatment (type/dose/frequency): ____________

Stretches (2-3 min. twice daily)	RV BTG, Words, etc. (2-3 min. twice daily)	RV Chant (1-2 min. daily)	RV Messa di voce (1-2 min. daily)	RV Vocal Communicator (throughout day)	RV Minis (throughout day)
AM					
PM					

❑ RV BTG (Basic Training Gesture) = Sustain "mmmmm" on a comfortable pitch about 10 times.

❑ RV Words, Phrases, Scales = make up words starting with "nnnn"; "gegegege"; "rrrrr"; "llllll"; "zzzzz"; "vvvvv"; ngngngng"; "mmmm"

❑ RV Chant (first all on one pitch; then, repeat sentence with increasing inflection until you are on an RV "roll").: No no no no no no; no no to to no no; no no, Toto, no no! /zi zi zi zi zi zi; zi zi si si zi zi/; Ziti Sissy, ziti! /vu vu vu vu vu vu; vu vu fu fu vu vu/; Voodoo, foolish voodoo!

❑ RV Vocal Communicator = "m-hmmm", "really", "right", "yeah", "no"

Do you feel vibrations? Is voice easy?

❑ RV Mini. "pull out" to RV; at phrase or other boundary, switch positions, take a breath, and come back in with strong RV:

Using a filled-in circle, indicate how your voice is today, overall, compared to when you first started therapy ("X" shows your rating at the start of therapy) (0 = catastrophic; 10 = exquisitely excellent).

	Start of Therapy	Today
10		
9		
8		
7		
6		
5		
4		
3		
2		
1		
0		

Other comments (successes, difficulties, etc.):____________

____

SESSIONS 3-4 HOME PROGRAM *YOU FILL OUT*

Date:____________________

Hydration Therapy

- ❑ Water intake daily (amount):____________________
- ❑ Steam or vapor (indicate type/number of times daily/duration): ____________________
- ❑ Medication (per your physician; type, dose, daily frequency):____________________

LPR

- ❑ Behavioral treatment
  - ◆ Reduce or eliminate spicy foods, alcohol, caffeine, and fatty foods
  - ◆ Engage in weight reduction program
  - ◆ Do not exercise immediately after eating
  - ◆ Elevate head of bed 6"
  - ◆ Do not eat for 3-4 hours before lying down
  - ◆ Do not smoke
- ❑ Drug treatment (type/dose/frequency):____________________

Stretches (2-3 min. twice daily)	RV BTG, Words, etc. (2-3 min. twice daily)	RV Chant (1-2 min. daily)	RV Messa di voce (1-2 min. daily)	RV Vocal Communicator (throughout day)	RV Minis (throughout day)
AM					
PM					

- ❑ RV BTG (Basic Training Gesture) = Sustain "mmmmm" on a comfortable pitch about 10 times.
- ❑ RV Words, Phrases, Scales = make up words starting with "nnnn";"gegegege";"rrrrr";"llllll"; "zzzzz";"vvvvv"; ngngngng";"mmmm"
- ❑ RV Chant (first all on one pitch; then, repeat sentence with increasing inflection until you are on an RV "roll").: No no no no no no; no no to to no no; no no, Toto, no no! /zi zi zi zi zi zi; zi zi si si zi zi/; Ziti Sissy, ziti! /vu vu vu vu vu vu; vu vu fu fu vu vu/; Voodoo, foolish voodoo!
- ❑ RV Vocal Communicator = "m-hmmm", "really", "right", "yeah", "no"
- ❑ RV Mini. "pull out" to RV; at phrase or other boundary, switch positions, take a breath, and come back in with strong RV:

Do you feel vibrations? Is voice easy?

Using a filled-in circle, indicate how your voice is today, overall, compared to when you first started therapy ("X" shows your rating at the start of therapy) (0 = catastrophic; 10 = exquisitely excellent).

	Start of Therapy	**Today**
10		
9		
8		
7		
6		
5		
4		
3		
2		
1		
0		

Other comments (successes, difficulties, etc.):____________________

If Sessions 5 and 6 are conducted on the same day, use the sheets for Session 5 only and omit Session 6 exercises from the home program.

SESSIONS 5-6 HOME PROGRAM **TEMPLATE**

Date: ____________________

Hydration Therapy

❑ Water intake daily (amount): ____________________

❑ Steam or vapor (indicate type/number of times daily/duration): ____________________

❑ Medication (per your physician; type, dose, daily frequency): ____________________

LPR

❑ Behavioral treatment
- ◆ Reduce or eliminate spicy foods, alcohol, caffeine, and fatty foods
- ◆ Engage in weight reduction program
- ◆ Do not exercise immediately after eating
- ◆ Elevate head of bed 6"
- ◆ Do not eat for 3-4 hours before lying down
- ◆ Do not smoke

❑ Drug treatment (type/dose/frequency): ____________________

Stretches (2-3 min. twice daily)	RV BTG, Words, etc. (2-3 min. twice daily)	RV Chant (1-2 min. daily)	RV Messa di voce (1-2 min. daily)	RV Vocal Communicator (throughout day)	RV Minis (throughout day)
AM					
PM					

❑ RV BTG (Basic Training Gesture) = Sustain "mmmmm" on a comfortable pitch about 10 times.

❑ RV Words, Phrases, Scales = make up words starting with "nnnn";"gegegege";"rrrrr";"llllll"; "zzzzz";"vvvvv"; ngngngng";"mmmm"

❑ RV Messa di voce: start with quietest, pinpoint RV; grow louder evenly over a count of 4, by "opening up,""strengthening sound in your face." Grow quieter evenly over a count of 4: "Hey, yo, hey Joe!"; dancing, rain, remain, zoo, verbal, love, swimming, vote, met, nanny, lawn, middle, near, zombie; zap, mate, singing, knock, romp, zone, meet, volume, tong, lamp, rest, victim, loop, nerd

❑ RV Vocal Communicator = "m-hmmm","really","right","yeah","no"

Do you feel vibrations? Is voice easy?

❑ RV Mini. "pull out" to RV; at phrase or other boundary, switch positions, take a breath, and come back in with strong RV

Using a filled-in circle, indicate how your voice is today, overall, compared to when you first started therapy ("X" shows your rating at the start of therapy) (0 = catastrophic; 10 = exquisitely excellent).

	Start of Therapy	Today
10		
9		
8		
7		
6		
5		
4		
3		
2		
1		
0		

Other comments (successes, difficulties, etc.): ____________________

SESSIONS 5-6 HOME PROGRAM *YOU FILL OUT* Date:________________

Hydration Therapy

❑ Water intake daily (amount):________________

❑ Steam or vapor (indicate type/number of times daily/duration): ________________

❑ Medication (per your physician; type, dose, daily frequency): ________________

LPR

❑ Behavioral treatment

- Reduce or eliminate spicy foods, alcohol, caffeine, and fatty foods
- Engage in weight reduction program
- Do not exercise immediately after eating
- Elevate head of bed 6"
- Do not eat for 3-4 hours before lying down
- Do not smoke

❑ Drug treatment (type/dose/frequency): ________________

Stretches (2-3 min. twice daily)	RV BTG, Words, etc. (2-3 min. twice daily)	RV Chant (1-2 min. daily)	RV Messa di voce (1-2 min. daily)	RV Vocal Communicator (throughout day)	RV Minis (throughout day)
AM					
PM					

❑ RV BTG (Basic Training Gesture) = Sustain "mmmmm" on a comfortable pitch about 10 times.

❑ RV Words, Phrases, Scales = make up words starting with "nnnn";"gegegege";"rrrrr";"llllll"; "zzzzz";"vvvvv"; ngngngng";"mmmm"

❑ RV Messa di voce: start with quietest, pinpoint RV; grow louder evenly over a count of 4, by "opening up,""strengthening sound in your face." Grow quieter evenly over a count of 4: "Hey, yo, hey Joe!"; dancing, rain, remain, zoo, verbal, love, swimming, vote, met, nanny, lawn, middle, near, zombie; zap, mate, singing, knock, romp, zone, meet, volume, tong, lamp, rest, victim, loop, nerd

Do you feel vibrations? Is voice easy?

❑ RV Vocal Communicator = "m-hmmm","really","right","yeah","no"

❑ RV Mini. "pull out" to RV; at phrase or other boundary, switch positions, take a breath, and come back in with strong RV

Using a filled-in circle, indicate how your voice is today, overall, compared to when you first started therapy ("X" shows your rating at the start of therapy) (0 = catastrophic; 10 = exquisitely excellent).

	Start of Therapy	**Today**
10		
9		
8		
7		
6		
5		
4		
3		
2		
1		
0		

Other comments (successes, difficulties, etc.):________________

SESSIONS 5-6 HOME PROGRAM *YOU FILL OUT*

Date:_______________

Hydration Therapy

❑ Water intake daily (amount):_______________

❑ Steam or vapor (indicate type/number of times daily/duration): _______________

❑ Medication (per your physician; type, dose, daily frequency):_______________

LPR

❑ Behavioral treatment
- ◆ Reduce or eliminate spicy foods, alcohol, caffeine, and fatty foods
- ◆ Engage in weight reduction program
- ◆ Do not exercise immediately after eating
- ◆ Elevate head of bed 6"
- ◆ Do not eat for 3-4 hours before lying down
- ◆ Do not smoke

❑ Drug treatment (type/dose/frequency): _______________

Stretches (2-3 min. twice daily)	RV BTG, Words, etc. (2-3 min. twice daily)	RV Chant (1-2 min. daily)	RV Messa di voce (1-2 min. daily)	RV Vocal Communicator (throughout day)	RV Minis (throughout day)
AM					
PM					

❑ RV BTG (Basic Training Gesture) = Sustain "mmmmm" on a comfortable pitch about 10 times.

❑ RV Words, Phrases, Scales = make up words starting with "nnnn";"gegegege";"rrrrr";"lllll"; "zzzzz";"vvvvv"; ngngngng";"mmmm"

❑ RV Messa di voce: start with quietest, pinpoint RV; grow louder evenly over a count of 4, by "opening up,""strengthening sound in your face." Grow quieter evenly over a count of 4: "Hey, yo, hey Joe!"; dancing, rain, remain, zoo, verbal, love, swimming, vote, met, nanny, lawn, middle, near, zombie; zap, mate, singing, knock, romp, zone, meet, volume, tong, lamp, rest, victim, loop, nerd

Do you feel vibrations? Is voice easy?

❑ RV Vocal Communicator = "m-hmmm","really","right","yeah","no"

❑ RV Mini. "pull out" to RV; at phrase or other boundary, switch positions, take a breath, and come back in with strong RV

Using a filled-in circle, indicate how your voice is today, overall, compared to when you first started therapy ("X" shows your rating at the start of therapy) (0 = catastrophic; 10 = exquisitely excellent).

	Start of Therapy	Today
10		
9		
8		
7		
6		
5		
4		
3		
2		
1		
0		

Other comments (successes, difficulties, etc.):_______________

SESSIONS 5-6 HOME PROGRAM *YOU FILL OUT* Date:____________

Hydration Therapy

❑ Water intake daily (amount):____________

❑ Steam or vapor (indicate type/number of times daily/duration): ____________

❑ Medication (per your physician; type, dose, daily frequency): ____________

LPR

❑ Behavioral treatment

- ◆ Reduce or eliminate spicy foods, alcohol, caffeine, and fatty foods
- ◆ Engage in weight reduction program
- ◆ Do not exercise immediately after eating
- ◆ Elevate head of bed 6"
- ◆ Do not eat for 3-4 hours before lying down
- ◆ Do not smoke

❑ Drug treatment (type/dose/frequency): ____________

Stretches (2-3 min. twice daily)	RV BTG, Words, etc. (2-3 min. twice daily)	RV Chant (1-2 min. daily)	RV Messa di voce (1-2 min. daily)	RV Vocal Communicator (throughout day)	RV Minis (throughout day)
AM					
PM					

❑ RV BTG (Basic Training Gesture) = Sustain "mmmmm" on a comfortable pitch about 10 times.

❑ RV Words, Phrases, Scales = make up words starting with "nnnn";"gegegege";"rrrrr";"llllll"; "zzzzz";"vvvvv"; ngngngng";"mmmm"

❑ RV Messa di voce: start with quietest, pinpoint RV; grow louder evenly over a count of 4, by "opening up,""strengthening sound in your face." Grow quieter evenly over a count of 4: "Hey, yo, hey Joe!"; dancing, rain, remain, zoo, verbal, love, swimming, vote, met, nanny, lawn, middle, near, zombie; zap, mate, singing, knock, romp, zone, meet, volume, tong, lamp, rest, victim, loop, nerd

Do you feel vibrations? Is voice easy?

❑ RV Vocal Communicator = "m-hmmm","really","right","yeah","no"

❑ RV Mini."pull out" to RV; at phrase or other boundary, switch positions, take a breath, and come back in with strong RV

Using a filled-in circle, indicate how your voice is today, overall, compared to when you first started therapy ("X" shows your rating at the start of therapy) (0 = catastrophic; 10 = exquisitely excellent).

	Start of Therapy	**Today**
10		
9		
8		
7		
6		
5		
4		
3		
2		
1		
0		

Other comments (successes, difficulties, etc.):____________

Sessions 5-6 Home Program *You Fill Out*

Date:________________

Hydration Therapy

- ☐ Water intake daily (amount):________________
- ☐ Steam or vapor (indicate type/number of times daily/duration): ________________
- ☐ Medication (per your physician; type, dose, daily frequency):________________

LPR

- ☐ Behavioral treatment
  - ◆ Reduce or eliminate spicy foods, alcohol, caffeine, and fatty foods
  - ◆ Engage in weight reduction program
  - ◆ Do not exercise immediately after eating
  - ◆ Elevate head of bed 6"
  - ◆ Do not eat for 3-4 hours before lying down
  - ◆ Do not smoke
- ☐ Drug treatment (type/dose/frequency): ________________

Stretches (2-3 min. twice daily)	RV BTG, Words, etc. (2-3 min. twice daily)	RV Chant (1-2 min. daily)	RV Messa di voce (1-2 min. daily)	RV Vocal Communicator (throughout day)	RV Minis (throughout day)
AM					
PM					

- ☐ RV BTG (Basic Training Gesture) = Sustain "mmmmm" on a comfortable pitch about 10 times.
- ☐ RV Words, Phrases, Scales = make up words starting with "nnnn";"gegegege";"rrrrr";"llllll"; "zzzzz";"vvvvv"; ngngngng";"mmmm"
- ☐ RV Messa di voce: start with quietest, pinpoint RV; grow louder evenly over a count of 4, by "opening up,""strengthening sound in your face." Grow quieter evenly over a count of 4: "Hey, yo, hey Joe!"; dancing, rain, remain, zoo, verbal, love, swimming, vote, met, nanny, lawn, middle, near, zombie; zap, mate, singing, knock, romp, zone, meet, volume, tong, lamp, rest, victim, loop, nerd
- ☐ RV Vocal Communicator = "m-hmmm","really","right","yeah","no"
- ☐ RV Mini. "pull out" to RV; at phrase or other boundary, switch positions, take a breath, and come back in with strong RV

Do you feel vibrations? Is voice easy?

Using a filled-in circle, indicate how your voice is today, overall, compared to when you first started therapy ("X" shows your rating at the start of therapy) (0 = catastrophic; 10 = exquisitely excellent).

	Start of Therapy	**Today**
10		
9		
8		
7		
6		
5		
4		
3		
2		
1		
0		

Other comments (successes, difficulties, etc.): ________________

Sessions 5-6 Home Program *You Fill Out* Date:________________

Hydration Therapy

- ❑ Water intake daily (amount):________________
- ❑ Steam or vapor (indicate type/number of times daily/duration): ________________
- ❑ Medication (per your physician; type, dose, daily frequency): ________________

LPR

- ❑ Behavioral treatment
  - ◆ Reduce or eliminate spicy foods, alcohol, caffeine, and fatty foods
  - ◆ Engage in weight reduction program
  - ◆ Do not exercise immediately after eating
  - ◆ Elevate head of bed 6"
  - ◆ Do not eat for 3-4 hours before lying down
  - ◆ Do not smoke
- ❑ Drug treatment (type/dose/frequency): ________________

Stretches (2-3 min. twice daily)	RV BTG, Words, etc. (2-3 min. twice daily)	RV Chant (1-2 min. daily)	RV Messa di voce (1-2 min. daily)	RV Vocal Communicator (throughout day)	RV Minis (throughout day)
AM					
PM					

- ❑ RV BTG (Basic Training Gesture) = Sustain "mmmmm" on a comfortable pitch about 10 times.
- ❑ RV Words, Phrases, Scales = make up words starting with "nnnn";"gegegege";"rrrrr";"llllll"; "zzzzz";"vvvvv"; ngngngng";"mmmm"
- ❑ RV Messa di voce: start with quietest, pinpoint RV; grow louder evenly over a count of 4, by "opening up,""strengthening sound in your face." Grow quieter evenly over a count of 4: "Hey, yo, hey Joe!"; dancing, rain, remain, zoo, verbal, love, swimming, vote, met, nanny, lawn, middle, near, zombie; zap, mate, singing, knock, romp, zone, meet, volume, tong, lamp, rest, victim, loop, nerd
- ❑ RV Vocal Communicator = "m-hmmm","really","right","yeah","no"
- ❑ RV Mini."pull out" to RV; at phrase or other boundary, switch positions,

Do you feel vibrations? Is voice easy?

	Start of Therapy	Today
10		
9		
8		
7		
6		
5		
4		
3		
2		
1		
0		

Other comments (successes, difficulties, etc.): ________________

Sessions 5-6 Home Program *You Fill Out* Date:________

Hydration Therapy

- ❑ Water intake daily (amount):________
- ❑ Steam or vapor (indicate type/number of times daily/duration): ________
- ❑ Medication (per your physician; type, dose, daily frequency):________

LPR

- ❑ Behavioral treatment
  - ◆ Reduce or eliminate spicy foods, alcohol, caffeine, and fatty foods
  - ◆ Engage in weight reduction program
  - ◆ Do not exercise immediately after eating
  - ◆ Elevate head of bed 6"
  - ◆ Do not eat for 3-4 hours before lying down
  - ◆ Do not smoke
- ❑ Drug treatment (type/dose/frequency):________

Stretches (2-3 min. twice daily)	RV BTG, Words, etc. (2-3 min. twice daily)	RV Chant (1-2 min. daily)	RV Messa di voce (1-2 min. daily)	RV Vocal Communicator (throughout day)	RV Minis (throughout day)
AM					
PM					

- ❑ RV BTG (Basic Training Gesture) = Sustain "mmmmm" on a comfortable pitch about 10 times.
- ❑ RV Words, Phrases, Scales = make up words starting with "nnnn";"gegegege";"rrrrr";"llllll"; "zzzzz";"vvvvv"; ngngngng";"mmmm"
- ❑ RV Messa di voce: start with quietest, pinpoint RV; grow louder evenly over a count of 4, by "opening up,""strengthening sound in your face." Grow quieter evenly over a count of 4: "Hey, yo, hey Joe!"; dancing, rain, remain, zoo, verbal, love, swimming, vote, met, nanny, lawn, middle, near, zombie; zap, mate, singing, knock, romp, zone, meet, volume, tong, lamp, rest, victim, loop, nerd
- ❑ RV Vocal Communicator = "m-hmmm","really","right","yeah","no"
- ❑ RV Mini. "pull out" to RV; at phrase or other boundary, switch positions, take a breath, and come back in with strong RV

Do you feel vibrations? Is voice easy?

Using a filled-in circle, indicate how your voice is today, overall, compared to when you first started therapy ("X" shows your rating at the start of therapy) (0 = catastrophic; 10 = exquisitely excellent).

	Start of Therapy	Today
10		
9		
8		
7		
6		
5		
4		
3		
2		
1		
0		

Other comments (successes, difficulties, etc.):________

SESSIONS 5-6 HOME PROGRAM ***YOU FILL OUT*** Date:________________

Hydration Therapy

❑ Water intake daily (amount):________________

❑ Steam or vapor (indicate type/number of times daily/duration): ________________

❑ Medication (per your physician; type, dose, daily frequency):________________

LPR

❑ Behavioral treatment

- ◆ Reduce or eliminate spicy foods, alcohol, caffeine, and fatty foods
- ◆ Engage in weight reduction program
- ◆ Do not exercise immediately after eating
- ◆ Elevate head of bed 6"
- ◆ Do not eat for 3-4 hours before lying down
- ◆ Do not smoke

❑ Drug treatment (type/dose/frequency):________________

Stretches (2-3 min. twice daily)	RV BTG, Words, etc. (2-3 min. twice daily)	RV Chant (1-2 min. daily)	RV Messa di voce (1-2 min. daily)	RV Vocal Communicator (throughout day)	RV Minis (throughout day)
AM					
PM					

❑ RV BTG (Basic Training Gesture) = Sustain "mmmmm" on a comfortable pitch about 10 times.

❑ RV Words, Phrases, Scales = make up words starting with "nnnn";"gegegege";"rrrrr";"llllll"; "zzzzz";"vvvvv"; ngngngng";"mmmm"

❑ RV Chant (first all on one pitch; then, repeat sentence with increasing inflection until you are on an RV "roll").: No no no no no no; no no to to no no; no no, Toto, no no! /zi zi zi zi zi zi; zi zi si si zi zi/; Ziti Sissy, ziti! /vu vu vu vu vu vu; vu vu fu fu vu vu/; Voodoo, foolish voodoo!

❑ RV Vocal Communicator = "m-hmmm","really","right","yeah","no"

Do you feel vibrations? Is voice easy?

❑ RV Mini. "pull out" to RV; at phrase or other boundary, switch positions, take a breath, and come back in with strong RV:

Using a filled-in circle, indicate how your voice is today, overall, compared to when you first started therapy ("X" shows your rating at the start of therapy) (0 = catastrophic; 10 = exquisitely excellent).

	Start of Therapy	**Today**
10		
9		
8		
7		
6		
5		
4		
3		
2		
1		
0		

Other comments (successes, difficulties, etc.):________________

SESSIONS 5-6 HOME PROGRAM *YOU FILL OUT*

Date:____________________

Hydration Therapy

- ❑ Water intake daily (amount):____________________
- ❑ Steam or vapor (indicate type/number of times daily/duration): ____________________
- ❑ Medication (per your physician; type, dose, daily frequency):____________________

LPR

- ❑ Behavioral treatment
  - ◆ Reduce or eliminate spicy foods, alcohol, caffeine, and fatty foods
  - ◆ Engage in weight reduction program
  - ◆ Do not exercise immediately after eating
  - ◆ Elevate head of bed 6"
  - ◆ Do not eat for 3-4 hours before lying down
  - ◆ Do not smoke
- ❑ Drug treatment (type/dose/frequency):____________________

Stretches (2-3 min. twice daily)	RV BTG, Words, etc. (2-3 min. twice daily)	RV Chant (1-2 min. daily)	RV Messa di voce (1-2 min. daily)	RV Vocal Communicator (throughout day)	RV Minis (throughout day)
AM					
PM					

- ❑ RV BTG (Basic Training Gesture) = Sustain "mmmmm" on a comfortable pitch about 10 times.
- ❑ RV Words, Phrases, Scales = make up words starting with "nnnn";"gegegege";"rrrrr";"llllll"; "zzzzz";"vvvvv"; ngngngng";"mmmm"
- ❑ RV Chant (first all on one pitch; then, repeat sentence with increasing inflection until you are on an RV "roll").: No no no no no no; no no to to no no; no no, Toto, no no! /zi zi zi zi zi zi; zi zi si si zi zi/; Ziti Sissy, ziti! /vu vu vu vu vu vu; vu vu fu fu vu vu/; Voodoo, foolish voodoo!
- ❑ RV Vocal Communicator = "m-hmmm", "really", "right", "yeah", "no"
- ❑ RV Mini. "pull out" to RV; at phrase or other boundary, switch positions, take a breath, and come back in with strong RV:

Do you feel vibrations? Is voice easy?

Using a filled-in circle, indicate how your voice is today, overall, compared to when you first started therapy ("X" shows your rating at the start of therapy) (0 = catastrophic; 10 = exquisitely excellent).

	Start of Therapy	**Today**
10		
9		
8		
7		
6		
5		
4		
3		
2		
1		
0		

Other comments (successes, difficulties, etc.):____________________

Sessions 5-6 Home Program *You Fill Out* Date:________________

Hydration Therapy

- ❑ Water intake daily (amount):________________
- ❑ Steam or vapor (indicate type/number of times daily/duration): ________________
- ❑ Medication (per your physician; type, dose, daily frequency):________________

LPR

- ❑ Behavioral treatment
  - ◆ Reduce or eliminate spicy foods, alcohol, caffeine, and fatty foods
  - ◆ Engage in weight reduction program
  - ◆ Do not exercise immediately after eating
  - ◆ Elevate head of bed 6"
  - ◆ Do not eat for 3-4 hours before lying down
  - ◆ Do not smoke
- ❑ Drug treatment (type/dose/frequency): ________________

Stretches (2-3 min. twice daily)	RV BTG, Words, etc. (2-3 min. twice daily)	RV Chant (1-2 min. daily)	RV Messa di voce (1-2 min. daily)	RV Vocal Communicator (throughout day)	RV Minis (throughout day)
AM					
PM					

- ❑ RV BTG (Basic Training Gesture) = Sustain "mmmmm" on a comfortable pitch about 10 times.
- ❑ RV Words, Phrases, Scales = make up words starting with "nnnn";"gegegege";"rrrrr";"lllll"; "zzzzz";"vvvvv"; ngngngng";"mmmm"
- ❑ RV Chant (first all on one pitch; then, repeat sentence with increasing inflection until you are on an RV "roll").: No no no no no no; no no to to no no; no no, Toto, no no! /zi zi zi zi zi zi; zi zi si si zi zi/; Ziti Sissy, ziti! /vu vu vu vu vu vu; vu vu fu fu vu vu/; Voodoo, foolish voodoo!
- ❑ RV Vocal Communicator = "m-hmmm", "really", "right", "yeah", "no"
- ❑ RV Mini. "pull out" to RV; at phrase or other boundary, switch positions, take a breath, and come back in with strong RV:

Do you feel vibrations? Is voice easy?

Using a filled-in circle, indicate how your voice is today, overall, compared to when you first started therapy ("X" shows your rating at the start of therapy) (0 = catastrophic; 10 = exquisitely excellent).

	Start of Therapy	Today
10		
9		
8		
7		
6		
5		
4		
3		
2		
1		
0		

Other comments (successes, difficulties, etc.):________________

____

SESSIONS 5-6 HOME PROGRAM *YOU FILL OUT*

Date:____________________

Hydration Therapy

- ❑ Water intake daily (amount):____________________
- ❑ Steam or vapor (indicate type/number of times daily/duration): ____________________
- ❑ Medication (per your physician; type, dose, daily frequency):____________________

LPR

- ❑ Behavioral treatment
  - ◆ Reduce or eliminate spicy foods, alcohol, caffeine, and fatty foods
  - ◆ Engage in weight reduction program
  - ◆ Do not exercise immediately after eating
  - ◆ Elevate head of bed 6"
  - ◆ Do not eat for 3-4 hours before lying down
  - ◆ Do not smoke
- ❑ Drug treatment (type/dose/frequency): ____________________

Stretches (2-3 min. twice daily)	RV BTG, Words, etc. (2-3 min. twice daily)	RV Chant (1-2 min. daily)	RV Messa di voce (1-2 min. daily)	RV Vocal Communicator (throughout day)	RV Minis (throughout day)
AM					
PM					

- ❑ RV BTG (Basic Training Gesture) = Sustain "mmmmm" on a comfortable pitch about 10 times.
- ❑ RV Words, Phrases, Scales = make up words starting with "nnnn";"gegegege";"rrrrr";"llllll"; "zzzzz";"vvvvv"; ngngngng";"mmmm"
- ❑ RV Chant (first all on one pitch; then, repeat sentence with increasing inflection until you are on an RV "roll").: No no no no no no; no no to to no no; no no, Toto, no no! /zi zi zi zi zi zi; zi zi si si zi zi/; Ziti Sissy, ziti! /vu vu vu vu vu vu; vu vu fu fu vu vu/; Voodoo, foolish voodoo!
- ❑ RV Vocal Communicator = "m-hmmm", "really", "right", "yeah", "no"
- ❑ RV Mini. "pull out" to RV; at phrase or other boundary, switch positions, take a breath, and come back in with strong RV:

Do you feel vibrations? Is voice easy?

Using a filled-in circle, indicate how your voice is today, overall, compared to when you first started therapy ("X" shows your rating at the start of therapy) (0 = catastrophic; 10 = exquisitely excellent).

	Start of Therapy	Today
10		
9		
8		
7		
6		
5		
4		
3		
2		
1		
0		

Other comments (successes, difficulties, etc.):____________________

____

HOME PROGRAM *YOU FILL OUT*

Date:________________

Hydration Therapy

❑ Water intake daily (amount):________________

❑ Steam or vapor (indicate type/number of times daily/duration): ________________

❑ Medication (per your physician; type, dose, daily frequency):________________

LPR

❑ Behavioral treatment

- Reduce or eliminate spicy foods, alcohol, caffeine, and fatty foods
- Engage in weight reduction program
- Do not exercise immediately after eating
- Elevate head of bed 6"
- Do not eat for 3-4 hours before lying down
- Do not smoke

❑ Drug treatment (type/dose/frequency):________________

Stretches (2-3 min. twice daily)	RV BTG, Words, etc. (2-3 min. twice daily)	RV Chant (1-2 min. daily)	RV Messa di voce (1-2 min. daily)	RV Vocal Communicator (throughout day)	RV Minis (throughout day)
AM					
PM					

❑ RV BTG (Basic Training Gesture) = Sustain "mmmmm" on a comfortable pitch about 10 times.

❑ RV Words, Phrases, Scales = make up words starting with "nnnn";"gegegege";"rrrrr";"lllll"; "zzzzz";"vvvvv"; ngngngng";"mmmm"

❑ RV Chant (first all on one pitch; then, repeat sentence with increasing inflection until you are on an RV "roll").: No no no no no no; no no to to no no; no no, Toto, no no! /zi zi zi zi zi zi; zi zi si si zi zi/; Ziti Sissy, ziti! /vu vu vu vu vu vu; vu vu fu fu vu vu/; Voodoo, foolish voodoo!

❑ RV Vocal Communicator = "m-hmmm", "really", "right", "yeah", "no"

Do you feel vibrations? Is voice easy?

❑ RV Mini. "pull out" to RV; at phrase or other boundary, switch positions, take a breath, and come back in with strong RV:

Using a filled-in circle, indicate how your voice is today, overall, compared to when you first started therapy ("X" shows your rating at the start of therapy) (0 = catastrophic; 10 = exquisitely excellent).

	Start of Therapy	**Today**
10		
9		
8		
7		
6		
5		
4		
3		
2		
1		
0		

Other comments (successes, difficulties, etc.):________________

____

Sessions 5-6 Home Program *You Fill Out*

Date:______________

Hydration Therapy

❑ Water intake daily (amount):______________

❑ Steam or vapor (indicate type/number of times daily/duration): ______________

❑ Medication (per your physician; type, dose, daily frequency):______________

LPR

❑ Behavioral treatment

- Reduce or eliminate spicy foods, alcohol, caffeine, and fatty foods
- Engage in weight reduction program
- Do not exercise immediately after eating
- Elevate head of bed 6"
- Do not eat for 3-4 hours before lying down
- Do not smoke

❑ Drug treatment (type/dose/frequency):______________

Stretches (2-3 min. twice daily)	RV BTG, Words, etc. (2-3 min. twice daily)	RV Chant (1-2 min. daily)	RV Messa di voce (1-2 min. daily)	RV Vocal Communicator (throughout day)	RV Minis (throughout day)
AM					
PM					

❑ RV BTG (Basic Training Gesture) = Sustain "mmmmm" on a comfortable pitch about 10 times.

❑ RV Words, Phrases, Scales = make up words starting with "nnnn";"gegegege";"rrrrr";"llllll"; "zzzzz";"vvvvv"; ngngngng";"mmmm"

❑ RV Chant (first all on one pitch; then, repeat sentence with increasing inflection until you are on an RV "roll").: No no no no no no; no no to to no no; no no,Toto, no no! /zi zi zi zi zi zi; zi zi si si zi zi/; Ziti Sissy, ziti! /vu vu vu vu vu vu; vu vu fu fu vu vu/; Voodoo, foolish voodoo!

Do you feel vibrations? Is voice easy?

❑ RV Vocal Communicator = "m-hmmm","really","right","yeah","no"

❑ RV Mini."pull out" to RV; at phrase or other boundary, switch positions, take a breath, and come back in with strong RV:

Using a filled-in circle, indicate how your voice is today, overall, compared to when you first started therapy ("X" shows your rating at the start of therapy) (0 = catastrophic; 10 = exquisitely excellent).

	Start of Therapy	Today
10		
9		
8		
7		
6		
5		
4		
3		
2		
1		
0		

Other comments (successes, difficulties, etc.):______________

Sessions 5-6 Home Program *You Fill Out* Date:__________

Hydration Therapy

- ❑ Water intake daily (amount): __________
- ❑ Steam or vapor (indicate type/number of times daily/duration): __________
- ❑ Medication (per your physician; type, dose, daily frequency): __________

LPR

- ❑ Behavioral treatment
  - ◆ Reduce or eliminate spicy foods, alcohol, caffeine, and fatty foods
  - ◆ Engage in weight reduction program
  - ◆ Do not exercise immediately after eating
  - ◆ Elevate head of bed 6”
  - ◆ Do not eat for 3-4 hours before lying down
  - ◆ Do not smoke
- ❑ Drug treatment (type/dose/frequency): __________

Stretches (2-3 min. twice daily)	RV BTG, Words, etc. (2-3 min. twice daily)	RV Chant (1-2 min. daily)	RV Messa di voce (1-2 min. daily)	RV Vocal Communicator (throughout day)	RV Minis (throughout day)
AM					
PM					

- ❑ RV BTG (Basic Training Gesture) = Sustain “mmmmm” on a comfortable pitch about 10 times.
- ❑ RV Words, Phrases, Scales = make up words starting with “nnnn”; “gegegege”; “rrrrr”; “llllll”; “zzzzz”; “vvvvv”; ngngngng”; “mmmm”
- ❑ RV Chant (first all on one pitch; then, repeat sentence with increasing inflection until you are on an RV “roll”).: No no no no no no; no no to to no no; no no, Toto, no no! /zi zi zi zi zi zi; zi zi si si zi zi/; Ziti Sissy, ziti! /vu vu vu vu vu vu; vu vu fu fu vu vu/; Voodoo, foolish voodoo!
- ❑ RV Vocal Communicator = “m-hmmm”, “really”, “right”, “yeah”, “no”
- ❑ RV Mini. “pull out” to RV; at phrase or other boundary, switch positions, take a breath, and come back in with strong RV:

Do you feel vibrations? Is voice easy?

Using a filled-in circle, indicate how your voice is today, overall, compared to when you first started therapy (“X” shows your rating at the start of therapy) (0 = catastrophic; 10 = exquisitely excellent).

	Start of Therapy	Today
10		
9		
8		
7		
6		
5		
4		
3		
2		
1		
0		

Other comments (successes, difficulties, etc.): __________

Sessions 5-6 — Home Program *You Fill Out*

Date:____________________

Hydration Therapy

- ❑ Water intake daily (amount):____________________
- ❑ Steam or vapor (indicate type/number of times daily/duration): ____________________
- ❑ Medication (per your physician; type, dose, daily frequency):____________________

LPR

- ❑ Behavioral treatment
  - ◆ Reduce or eliminate spicy foods, alcohol, caffeine, and fatty foods
  - ◆ Engage in weight reduction program
  - ◆ Do not exercise immediately after eating
  - ◆ Elevate head of bed 6"
  - ◆ Do not eat for 3-4 hours before lying down
  - ◆ Do not smoke
- ❑ Drug treatment (type/dose/frequency):____________________

Stretches (2-3 min. twice daily)	RV BTG, Words, etc. (2-3 min. twice daily)	RV Chant (1-2 min. daily)	RV Messa di voce (1-2 min. daily)	RV Vocal Communicator (throughout day)	RV Minis (throughout day)
AM					
PM					

- ❑ RV BTG (Basic Training Gesture) = Sustain "mmmmm" on a comfortable pitch about 10 times.
- ❑ RV Words, Phrases, Scales = make up words starting with "nnnn";"gegegege";"rrrrr";"llllll"; "zzzzz";"vvvvv"; ngngngng";"mmmm"
- ❑ RV Chant (first all on one pitch; then, repeat sentence with increasing inflection until you are on an RV "roll").: No no no no no no; no no to to no no; no no, Toto, no no! /zi zi zi zi zi zi; zi zi si si zi zi/; Ziti Sissy, ziti! /vu vu vu vu vu vu; vu vu fu fu vu vu/; Voodoo, foolish voodoo!
- ❑ RV Vocal Communicator = "m-hmmm", "really", "right", "yeah", "no"
- ❑ RV Mini. "pull out" to RV; at phrase or other boundary, switch positions, take a breath, and come back in with strong RV:

Do you feel vibrations? Is voice easy?

Using a filled-in circle, indicate how your voice is today, overall, compared to when you first started therapy ("X" shows your rating at the start of therapy) (0 = catastrophic; 10 = exquisitely excellent).

	Start of Therapy	**Today**
10		
9		
8		
7		
6		
5		
4		
3		
2		
1		
0		

Other comments (successes, difficulties, etc.):____________________

If Sessions 7 and 8 are conducted on the same day, proceed immediately to discharge program.

SESSIONS 7-8 HOME PROGRAM TEMPLATE

Date: ______________________

Hydration Therapy

❑ Water intake daily (amount): ______________________

❑ Steam or vapor (indicate type/number of times daily/duration): ______________________

❑ Medication (per your physician; type, dose, daily frequency): ______________________

LPR

❑ Behavioral treatment

- ◆ Reduce or eliminate spicy foods, alcohol, caffeine, and fatty foods
- ◆ Engage in weight reduction program
- ◆ Do not exercise immediately after eating
- ◆ Elevate head of bed 6"
- ◆ Do not eat for 3-4 hours before lying down
- ◆ Do not smoke

❑ Drug treatment (type/dose/frequency): ______________________

Stretches (2-3 min. twice daily)	RV BTG, Words, etc. (2-3 min. twice daily)	RV Chant (1-2 min. daily)	RV Messa di voce (1-2 min. daily)	RV Vocal Communicator (throughout day)	RV Minis (throughout day)
AM					
PM					

❑ RV BTG (Basic Training Gesture) = Sustain "mmmmm" on a comfortable pitch about 10 times.

❑ RV Words, Phrases, Scales = make up words starting with "nnnn"; "gegegege"; "rrrrr"; "lllll"; "zzzzz"; "vvvvv"; ngngngng"; "mmmm"

Do you feel vibrations? Is voice easy?

❑ RV Messa di voce: start with quietest, pinpoint RV; grow louder evenly over a count of 4, by "opening up," "strengthening sound in your face." Grow quieter evenly over a count of 4: "Hey, yo, hey Joe!"; zebra, voodoo, working, Monday, lit, playing, vigor, rugged, nerve, zodiac, nonsense, metal, log, race

Using a filled-in circle, indicate how your voice is today, overall, compared to when you first started therapy ("X" shows your rating at the start of therapy) (0 = catastrophic; 10 = exquisitely excellent).

	Start of Therapy	Today
10		
9		
8		
7		
6		
5		
4		
3		
2		
1		
0		

Other comments (successes, difficulties, etc.): ______________________

Sessions 7-8 Home Program *You Fill Out*

Date:__________________

Hydration Therapy

❑ Water intake daily (amount):____________________

❑ Steam or vapor (indicate type/number of times daily/duration): ____________________

❑ Medication (per your physician; type, dose, daily frequency): ____________________

LPR

❑ Behavioral treatment
- ◆ Reduce or eliminate spicy foods, alcohol, caffeine, and fatty foods
- ◆ Engage in weight reduction program
- ◆ Do not exercise immediately after eating
- ◆ Elevate head of bed 6"
- ◆ Do not eat for 3-4 hours before lying down
- ◆ Do not smoke

❑ Drug treatment (type/dose/frequency): ____________________

Stretches (2-3 min. twice daily)	RV BTG, Words, etc. (2-3 min. twice daily)	RV Chant (1-2 min. daily)	RV Messa di voce (1-2 min. daily)	RV Vocal Communicator (throughout day)	RV Minis (throughout day)
AM					
PM					

❑ RV BTG (Basic Training Gesture) = Sustain "mmmmm" on a comfortable pitch about 10 times.

❑ RV Words, Phrases, Scales = make up words starting with "nnnn"; "gegegege";"rrrrr";"lllll";"zzzzz";"vvvvv"; ngngngng";"mmmm"

Do you feel vibrations? Is voice easy?

❑ RV Messa di voce: start with quietest, pinpoint RV; grow louder evenly over a count of 4, by "opening up,""strengthening sound in your face." Grow quieter evenly over a count of 4: "Hey, yo, hey Joe!"; zebra, voodoo, working, Monday, lit, playing, vigor, rugged, nerve, zodiac, nonsense, metal, log, race

Using a filled-in circle, indicate how your voice is today, overall, compared to when you first started therapy ("X" shows your rating at the start of therapy) (0 = catastrophic; 10 = exquisitely excellent).

	Start of Therapy	**Today**
10		
9		
8		
7		
6		
5		
4		
3		
2		
1		
0		

Other comments (successes, difficulties, etc.): ____________________

Sessions 7-8 Home Program *You Fill Out* Date:____________

Hydration Therapy

- ❑ Water intake daily (amount):____________
- ❑ Steam or vapor (indicate type/number of times daily/duration): ____________
- ❑ Medication (per your physician; type, dose, daily frequency):____________

LPR

- ❑ Behavioral treatment
  - ◆ Reduce or eliminate spicy foods, alcohol, caffeine, and fatty foods
  - ◆ Engage in weight reduction program
  - ◆ Do not exercise immediately after eating
  - ◆ Elevate head of bed 6"
  - ◆ Do not eat for 3-4 hours before lying down
  - ◆ Do not smoke
- ❑ Drug treatment (type/dose/frequency):____________

Stretches (2-3 min. twice daily)	RV BTG, Words, etc. (2-3 min. twice daily)	RV Chant (1-2 min. daily)	RV Messa di voce (1-2 min. daily)	RV Vocal Communicator (throughout day)	RV Minis (throughout day)
AM					
PM					

- ❑ RV BTG (Basic Training Gesture) = Sustain "mmmmm" on a comfortable pitch about 10 times.
- ❑ RV Words, Phrases, Scales = make up words starting with "nnnn"; "gegegege";"rrrrr";"lllll";"zzzzz";"vvvvv"; ngngngng";"mmmm"

Do you feel vibrations? Is voice easy?

- ❑ RV Messa di voce: start with quietest, pinpoint RV; grow louder evenly over a count of 4, by "opening up,""strengthening sound in your face." Grow quieter evenly over a count of 4: "Hey, yo, hey Joe!"; zebra, voodoo, working, Monday, lit, playing, vigor, rugged, nerve, zodiac, nonsense, metal, log, race

Using a filled-in circle, indicate how your voice is today, overall, compared to when you first started therapy ("X" shows your rating at the start of therapy) (0 = catastrophic; 10 = exquisitely excellent).

	Start of Therapy	Today
10		
9		
8		
7		
6		
5		
4		
3		
2		
1		
0		

Other comments (successes, difficulties, etc.):____________

SESSIONS 7-8 HOME PROGRAM *YOU FILL OUT* Date:__________________

Hydration Therapy

❑ Water intake daily (amount):______________________________

❑ Steam or vapor (indicate type/number of times daily/duration): ______________

❑ Medication (per your physician; type, dose, daily frequency):______________

LPR

❑ Behavioral treatment

- ◆ Reduce or eliminate spicy foods, alcohol, caffeine, and fatty foods
- ◆ Engage in weight reduction program
- ◆ Do not exercise immediately after eating
- ◆ Elevate head of bed 6"
- ◆ Do not eat for 3-4 hours before lying down
- ◆ Do not smoke

❑ Drug treatment (type/dose/frequency): ______________________

Stretches (2-3 min. twice daily)	RV BTG, Words, etc. (2-3 min. twice daily)	RV Chant (1-2 min. daily)	RV Messa di voce (1-2 min. daily)	RV Vocal Communicator (throughout day)	RV Minis (throughout day)
AM					
PM					

❑ RV BTG (Basic Training Gesture) = Sustain "mmmmm" on a comfortable pitch about 10 times.

❑ RV Words, Phrases, Scales = make up words starting with "nnnn"; "gegegege";"rrrrr";"lllll";"zzzzz";"vvvvv"; ngngngng";"mmmm"

Do you feel vibrations? Is voice easy?

❑ RV Messa di voce: start with quietest, pinpoint RV; grow louder evenly over a count of 4, by "opening up,""strengthening sound in your face." Grow quieter evenly over a count of 4: "Hey, yo, hey Joe!"; zebra, voodoo, working, Monday, lit, playing, vigor, rugged, nerve, zodiac, nonsense, metal, log, race

Using a filled-in circle, indicate how your voice is today, overall, compared to when you first started therapy ("X" shows your rating at the start of therapy) (0 = catastrophic; 10 = exquisitely excellent).

	Start of Therapy	Today
10		
9		
8		
7		
6		
5		
4		
3		
2		
1		
0		

Other comments (successes, difficulties, etc.):______________________

Sessions 7-8 Home Program *You Fill Out*

Date:__________________

Hydration Therapy

❑ Water intake daily (amount):__________________

❑ Steam or vapor (indicate type/number of times daily/duration): __________________

❑ Medication (per your physician; type, dose, daily frequency):__________________

LPR

❑ Behavioral treatment

- ◆ Reduce or eliminate spicy foods, alcohol, caffeine, and fatty foods
- ◆ Engage in weight reduction program
- ◆ Do not exercise immediately after eating
- ◆ Elevate head of bed 6"
- ◆ Do not eat for 3-4 hours before lying down
- ◆ Do not smoke

❑ Drug treatment (type/dose/frequency):__________________

Stretches (2-3 min. twice daily)	RV BTG, Words, etc. (2-3 min. twice daily)	RV Chant (1-2 min. daily)	RV Messa di voce (1-2 min. daily)	RV Vocal Communicator (throughout day)	RV Minis (throughout day)
AM					
PM					

❑ RV BTG (Basic Training Gesture) = Sustain "mmmmm" on a comfortable pitch about 10 times.

❑ RV Words, Phrases, Scales = make up words starting with "nnnn"; "gegegege";"rrrrr";"lllll";"zzzzz";"vvvvv"; ngngngng";"mmmm"

Do you feel vibrations? Is voice easy?

❑ RV Messa di voce: start with quietest, pinpoint RV; grow louder evenly over a count of 4, by "opening up,""strengthening sound in your face." Grow quieter evenly over a count of 4: "Hey, yo, hey Joe!"; zebra, voodoo, working, Monday, lit, playing, vigor, rugged, nerve, zodiac, nonsense, metal, log, race

Using a filled-in circle, indicate how your voice is today, overall, compared to when you first started therapy ("X" shows your rating at the start of therapy) (0 = catastrophic; 10 = exquisitely excellent).

	Start of Therapy	Today
10		
9		
8		
7		
6		
5		
4		
3		
2		
1		
0		

Other comments (successes, difficulties, etc.):__________________

SESSIONS 7-8 HOME PROGRAM *YOU FILL OUT* Date:____________

Hydration Therapy

❑ Water intake daily (amount):____________

❑ Steam or vapor (indicate type/number of times daily/duration): ____________

❑ Medication (per your physician; type, dose, daily frequency): ____________

LPR

❑ Behavioral treatment

- Reduce or eliminate spicy foods, alcohol, caffeine, and fatty foods
- Engage in weight reduction program
- Do not exercise immediately after eating
- Elevate head of bed 6"
- Do not eat for 3-4 hours before lying down
- Do not smoke

❑ Drug treatment (type/dose/frequency): ____________

Stretches (2-3 min. twice daily)	RV BTG, Words, etc. (2-3 min. twice daily)	RV Chant (1-2 min. daily)	RV Messa di voce (1-2 min. daily)	RV Vocal Communicator (throughout day)	RV Minis (throughout day)
AM					
PM					

❑ RV BTG (Basic Training Gesture) = Sustain "mmmmm" on a comfortable pitch about 10 times.

❑ RV Words, Phrases, Scales = make up words starting with "nnnn"; "gegegege";"rrrrr";"lllll";"zzzzz";"vvvvv"; ngngngng";"mmmm"

Do you feel vibrations? Is voice easy?

❑ RV Messa di voce: start with quietest, pinpoint RV; grow louder evenly over a count of 4, by "opening up,""strengthening sound in your face." Grow quieter evenly over a count of 4: "Hey, yo, hey Joe!"; zebra, voodoo, working, Monday, lit, playing, vigor, rugged, nerve, zodiac, nonsense, metal, log, race

Using a filled-in circle, indicate how your voice is today, overall, compared to when you first started therapy ("X" shows your rating at the start of therapy) (0 = catastrophic; 10 = exquisitely excellent).

	Start of Therapy	**Today**
10		
9		
8		
7		
6		
5		
4		
3		
2		
1		
0		

Other comments (successes, difficulties, etc.): ____________

Sessions 7-8 Home Program *You Fill Out*

Date:____________________

Hydration Therapy

- ❑ Water intake daily (amount):____________________
- ❑ Steam or vapor (indicate type/number of times daily/duration): ____________________
- ❑ Medication (per your physician; type, dose, daily frequency):____________________

LPR

- ❑ Behavioral treatment
  - ◆ Reduce or eliminate spicy foods, alcohol, caffeine, and fatty foods
  - ◆ Engage in weight reduction program
  - ◆ Do not exercise immediately after eating
  - ◆ Elevate head of bed 6"
  - ◆ Do not eat for 3-4 hours before lying down
  - ◆ Do not smoke
- ❑ Drug treatment (type/dose/frequency):____________________

Stretches (2-3 min. twice daily)	RV BTG, Words, etc. (2-3 min. twice daily)	RV Chant (1-2 min. daily)	RV Messa di voce (1-2 min. daily)	RV Vocal Communicator (throughout day)	RV Minis (throughout day)
AM					
PM					

- ❑ RV BTG (Basic Training Gesture) = Sustain "mmmmm" on a comfortable pitch about 10 times.
- ❑ RV Words, Phrases, Scales = make up words starting with "nnnn"; "gegegege";"rrrrr";"lllll";"zzzzz";"vvvvv"; ngngngng";"mmmm"

Do you feel vibrations? Is voice easy?

- ❑ RV Messa di voce: start with quietest, pinpoint RV; grow louder evenly over a count of 4, by "opening up,""strengthening sound in your face." Grow quieter evenly over a count of 4: "Hey, yo, hey Joe!"; zebra, voodoo, working, Monday, lit, playing, vigor, rugged, nerve, zodiac, nonsense, metal, log, race

Using a filled-in circle, indicate how your voice is today, overall, compared to when you first started therapy ("X" shows your rating at the start of therapy) (0 = catastrophic; 10 = exquisitely excellent).

	Start of Therapy	Today
10		
9		
8		
7		
6		
5		
4		
3		
2		
1		
0		

Other comments (successes, difficulties, etc.):____________________

SESSIONS 7-8   HOME PROGRAM ***YOU FILL OUT***   Date:____________

Hydration Therapy

- ❏ Water intake daily (amount):____________
- ❏ Steam or vapor (indicate type/number of times daily/duration): ____________
- ❏ Medication (per your physician; type, dose, daily frequency):____________

LPR

- ❏ Behavioral treatment
  - ◆ Reduce or eliminate spicy foods, alcohol, caffeine, and fatty foods
  - ◆ Engage in weight reduction program
  - ◆ Do not exercise immediately after eating
  - ◆ Elevate head of bed 6"
  - ◆ Do not eat for 3-4 hours before lying down
  - ◆ Do not smoke
- ❏ Drug treatment (type/dose/frequency):____________

Stretches (2-3 min. twice daily)	RV BTG, Words, etc. (2-3 min. twice daily)	RV Chant (1-2 min. daily)	RV Messa di voce (1-2 min. daily)	RV Vocal Communicator (throughout day)	RV Minis (throughout day)
AM					
PM					

- ❏ RV BTG (Basic Training Gesture) = Sustain "mmmmm" on a comfortable pitch about 10 times.
- ❏ RV Words, Phrases, Scales = make up words starting with "nnnn"; "gegegege";"rrrrr";"lllll";"zzzzz";"vvvvv"; ngngngng";"mmmm"

Do you feel vibrations? Is voice easy?

- ❏ RV Messa di voce: start with quietest, pinpoint RV; grow louder evenly over a count of 4, by "opening up,""strengthening sound in your face." Grow quieter evenly over a count of 4: "Hey, yo, hey Joe!"; zebra, voodoo, working, Monday, lit, playing, vigor, rugged, nerve, zodiac, nonsense, metal, log, race

Using a filled-in circle, indicate how your voice is today, overall, compared to when you first started therapy ("X" shows your rating at the start of therapy) (0 = catastrophic; 10 = exquisitely excellent).

	Start of Therapy	**Today**
10		
9		
8		
7		
6		
5		
4		
3		
2		
1		
0		

Other comments (successes, difficulties, etc.):____________

____

Sessions 7-8 Home Program *You Fill Out* Date:____________

Hydration Therapy

- ❑ Water intake daily (amount):____________
- ❑ Steam or vapor (indicate type/number of times daily/duration): ____________
- ❑ Medication (per your physician; type, dose, daily frequency):____________

LPR

- ❑ Behavioral treatment
  - ◆ Reduce or eliminate spicy foods, alcohol, caffeine, and fatty foods
  - ◆ Engage in weight reduction program
  - ◆ Do not exercise immediately after eating
  - ◆ Elevate head of bed 6"
  - ◆ Do not eat for 3-4 hours before lying down
  - ◆ Do not smoke
- ❑ Drug treatment (type/dose/frequency):____________

Stretches (2-3 min. twice daily)	RV BTG, Words, etc. (2-3 min. twice daily)	RV Chant (1-2 min. daily)	RV Messa di voce (1-2 min. daily)	RV Vocal Communicator (throughout day)	RV Minis (throughout day)
AM					
PM					

❑ RV BTG (Basic Training Gesture) = Sustain "mmmmm" on a comfortable pitch about 10 times.

❑ RV Words, Phrases, Scales = make up words starting with "nnnn"; "gegegege";"rrrrr";"lllll";"zzzzz";"vvvvv"; ngngngng";"mmmm"

Do you feel vibrations? Is voice easy?

❑ RV Messa di voce: start with quietest, pinpoint RV; grow louder evenly over a count of 4, by "opening up," "strengthening sound in your face." Grow quieter evenly over a count of 4: "Hey, yo, hey Joe!"; zebra, voodoo, working, Monday, lit, playing, vigor, rugged, nerve, zodiac, nonsense, metal, log, race

Using a filled-in circle, indicate how your voice is today, overall, compared to when you first started therapy ("X" shows your rating at the start of therapy) (0 = catastrophic; 10 = exquisitely excellent).

	Start of Therapy	Today
10		
9		
8		
7		
6		
5		
4		
3		
2		
1		
0		

Other comments (successes, difficulties, etc.):____________

Sessions 7-8 Home Program *You Fill Out*

Date:______________

Hydration Therapy

❑ Water intake daily (amount):______________

❑ Steam or vapor (indicate type/number of times daily/duration): ______________

❑ Medication (per your physician; type, dose, daily frequency): ______________

LPR

❑ Behavioral treatment

- Reduce or eliminate spicy foods, alcohol, caffeine, and fatty foods
- Engage in weight reduction program
- Do not exercise immediately after eating
- Elevate head of bed 6"
- Do not eat for 3-4 hours before lying down
- Do not smoke

❑ Drug treatment (type/dose/frequency): ______________

Stretches (2-3 min. twice daily)	RV BTG, Words, etc. (2-3 min. twice daily)	RV Chant (1-2 min. daily)	RV Messa di voce (1-2 min. daily)	RV Vocal Communicator (throughout day)	RV Minis (throughout day)
AM					
PM					

❑ RV BTG (Basic Training Gesture) = Sustain "mmmmm" on a comfortable pitch about 10 times.

❑ RV Words, Phrases, Scales = make up words starting with "nnnn"; "gegegege";"rrrrr";"llllll";"zzzzz";"vvvvv"; ngngngng";"mmmm"

Do you feel vibrations? Is voice easy?

❑ RV Messa di voce: start with quietest, pinpoint RV; grow louder evenly over a count of 4, by "opening up,""strengthening sound in your face." Grow quieter evenly over a count of 4: "Hey, yo, hey Joe!"; zebra, voodoo, working, Monday, lit, playing, vigor, rugged, nerve, zodiac, nonsense, metal, log, race

Using a filled-in circle, indicate how your voice is today, overall, compared to when you first started therapy ("X" shows your rating at the start of therapy) (0 = catastrophic; 10 = exquisitely excellent).

	Start of Therapy	Today
10		
9		
8		
7		
6		
5		
4		
3		
2		
1		
0		

Other comments (successes, difficulties, etc.): ______________

Sessions 7-8 Home Program *You Fill Out* Date:________________

Hydration Therapy

❑ Water intake daily (amount):________________

❑ Steam or vapor (indicate type/number of times daily/duration): ________________

❑ Medication (per your physician; type, dose, daily frequency):________________

LPR

❑ Behavioral treatment
- ◆ Reduce or eliminate spicy foods, alcohol, caffeine, and fatty foods
- ◆ Engage in weight reduction program
- ◆ Do not exercise immediately after eating
- ◆ Elevate head of bed 6"
- ◆ Do not eat for 3-4 hours before lying down
- ◆ Do not smoke

❑ Drug treatment (type/dose/frequency):________________

Stretches (2-3 min. twice daily)	RV BTG, Words, etc. (2-3 min. twice daily)	RV Chant (1-2 min. daily)	RV Messa di voce (1-2 min. daily)	RV Vocal Communicator (throughout day)	RV Minis (throughout day)
AM					
PM					

❑ RV BTG (Basic Training Gesture) = Sustain "mmmmm" on a comfortable pitch about 10 times.

❑ RV Words, Phrases, Scales = make up words starting with "nnnn"; "gegegege";"rrrrr";"lllll";"zzzzz";"vvvvv"; ngngngng";"mmmm"

Do you feel vibrations? Is voice easy?

❑ RV Messa di voce: start with quietest, pinpoint RV; grow louder evenly over a count of 4, by "opening up," "strengthening sound in your face." Grow quieter evenly over a count of 4: "Hey, yo, hey Joe!"; zebra, voodoo, working, Monday, lit, playing, vigor, rugged, nerve, zodiac, nonsense, metal, log, race

Using a filled-in circle, indicate how your voice is today, overall, compared to when you first started therapy ("X" shows your rating at the start of therapy) (0 = catastrophic; 10 = exquisitely excellent).

	Start of Therapy	**Today**
10		
9		
8		
7		
6		
5		
4		
3		
2		
1		
0		

Other comments (successes, difficulties, etc.):________________

SESSIONS 7-8 HOME PROGRAM *YOU FILL OUT* Date:____________

Hydration Therapy

❑ Water intake daily (amount):____________

❑ Steam or vapor (indicate type/number of times daily/duration): ____________

❑ Medication (per your physician; type, dose, daily frequency): ____________

LPR

❑ Behavioral treatment
- ◆ Reduce or eliminate spicy foods, alcohol, caffeine, and fatty foods
- ◆ Engage in weight reduction program
- ◆ Do not exercise immediately after eating
- ◆ Elevate head of bed 6"
- ◆ Do not eat for 3-4 hours before lying down
- ◆ Do not smoke

❑ Drug treatment (type/dose/frequency): ____________

Stretches (2-3 min. twice daily)	RV BTG, Words, etc. (2-3 min. twice daily)	RV Chant (1-2 min. daily)	RV Messa di voce (1-2 min. daily)	RV Vocal Communicator (throughout day)	RV Minis (throughout day)
AM					
PM					

❑ RV BTG (Basic Training Gesture) = Sustain "mmmmm" on a comfortable pitch about 10 times.

❑ RV Words, Phrases, Scales = make up words starting with "nnnn"; "gegegege";"rrrrr";"lllll";"zzzzz";"vvvvv"; ngngngng";"mmmm"

Do you feel vibrations?
Is voice easy?

❑ RV Messa di voce: start with quietest, pinpoint RV; grow louder evenly over a count of 4, by "opening up," "strengthening sound in your face." Grow quieter evenly over a count of 4: "Hey, yo, hey Joe!"; zebra, voodoo, working, Monday, lit, playing, vigor, rugged, nerve, zodiac, nonsense, metal, log, race

Using a filled-in circle, indicate how your voice is today, overall, compared to when you first started therapy ("X" shows your rating at the start of therapy) (0 = catastrophic; 10 = exquisitely excellent).

	Start of Therapy	**Today**
10		
9		
8		
7		
6		
5		
4		
3		
2		
1		
0		

Other comments (successes, difficulties, etc.): ____________

____

Sessions 7-8 Home Program *You Fill Out*

Date:________________

Hydration Therapy

- ❑ Water intake daily (amount):________________
- ❑ Steam or vapor (indicate type/number of times daily/duration): ________________
- ❑ Medication (per your physician; type, dose, daily frequency):________________

LPR

- ❑ Behavioral treatment
  - ◆ Reduce or eliminate spicy foods, alcohol, caffeine, and fatty foods
  - ◆ Engage in weight reduction program
  - ◆ Do not exercise immediately after eating
  - ◆ Elevate head of bed 6"
  - ◆ Do not eat for 3-4 hours before lying down
  - ◆ Do not smoke
- ❑ Drug treatment (type/dose/frequency):________________

Stretches (2-3 min. twice daily)	RV BTG, Words, etc. (2-3 min. twice daily)	RV Chant (1-2 min. daily)	RV Messa di voce (1-2 min. daily)	RV Vocal Communicator (throughout day)	RV Minis (throughout day)
AM					
PM					

❑ RV BTG (Basic Training Gesture) = Sustain "mmmmm" on a comfortable pitch about 10 times.

❑ RV Words, Phrases, Scales = make up words starting with "nnnn"; "gegegege"; "rrrrr"; "lllll"; "zzzzz"; "vvvvv"; ngngngng"; "mmmm"

Do you feel vibrations? Is voice easy?

❑ RV Messa di voce: start with quietest, pinpoint RV; grow louder evenly over a count of 4, by "opening up," "strengthening sound in your face." Grow quieter evenly over a count of 4: "Hey, yo, hey Joe!"; zebra, voodoo, working, Monday, lit, playing, vigor, rugged, nerve, zodiac, nonsense, metal, log, race

Using a filled-in circle, indicate how your voice is today, overall, compared to when you first started therapy ("X" shows your rating at the start of therapy) (0 = catastrophic; 10 = exquisitely excellent).

	Start of Therapy	Today
10		
9		
8		
7		
6		
5		
4		
3		
2		
1		
0		

Other comments (successes, difficulties, etc.):________________

SESSIONS 7-8 HOME PROGRAM *YOU FILL OUT* Date:__________

Hydration Therapy

- ❑ Water intake daily (amount):__________
- ❑ Steam or vapor (indicate type/number of times daily/duration): __________
- ❑ Medication (per your physician; type, dose, daily frequency):__________

LPR

- ❑ Behavioral treatment
  - ◆ Reduce or eliminate spicy foods, alcohol, caffeine, and fatty foods
  - ◆ Engage in weight reduction program
  - ◆ Do not exercise immediately after eating
  - ◆ Elevate head of bed 6"
  - ◆ Do not eat for 3-4 hours before lying down
  - ◆ Do not smoke
- ❑ Drug treatment (type/dose/frequency): __________

Stretches (2-3 min. twice daily)	RV BTG, Words, etc. (2-3 min. twice daily)	RV Chant (1-2 min. daily)	RV Messa di voce (1-2 min. daily)	RV Vocal Communicator (throughout day)	RV Minis (throughout day)
AM					
PM					

❑ RV BTG (Basic Training Gesture) = Sustain "mmmmm" on a comfortable pitch about 10 times.

❑ RV Words, Phrases, Scales = make up words starting with "nnnn"; "gegegege";"rrrrr";"llllll";"zzzzz";"vvvvv"; ngngngng";"mmmm"

Do you feel vibrations? Is voice easy?

❑ RV Messa di voce: start with quietest, pinpoint RV; grow louder evenly over a count of 4, by "opening up,""strengthening sound in your face." Grow quieter evenly over a count of 4: "Hey, yo, hey Joe!"; zebra, voodoo, working, Monday, lit, playing, vigor, rugged, nerve, zodiac, nonsense, metal, log, race

Using a filled-in circle, indicate how your voice is today, overall, compared to when you first started therapy ("X" shows your rating at the start of therapy) (0 = catastrophic; 10 = exquisitely excellent).

	Start of Therapy	Today
10		
9		
8		
7		
6		
5		
4		
3		
2		
1		
0		

Other comments (successes, difficulties, etc.):__________

SESSIONS 7-8 HOME PROGRAM *YOU FILL OUT* Date:______________

Hydration Therapy

- ❑ Water intake daily (amount):______________
- ❑ Steam or vapor (indicate type/number of times daily/duration): ______________
- ❑ Medication (per your physician; type, dose, daily frequency):______________

LPR

- ❑ Behavioral treatment
  - ◆ Reduce or eliminate spicy foods, alcohol, caffeine, and fatty foods
  - ◆ Engage in weight reduction program
  - ◆ Do not exercise immediately after eating
  - ◆ Elevate head of bed 6"
  - ◆ Do not eat for 3-4 hours before lying down
  - ◆ Do not smoke
- ❑ Drug treatment (type/dose/frequency):______________

Stretches (2-3 min. twice daily)	RV BTG, Words, etc. (2-3 min. twice daily)	RV Chant (1-2 min. daily)	RV Messa di voce (1-2 min. daily)	RV Vocal Communicator (throughout day)	RV Minis (throughout day)
AM					
PM					

- ❑ RV BTG (Basic Training Gesture) = Sustain "mmmmm" on a comfortable pitch about 10 times.
- ❑ RV Words, Phrases, Scales = make up words starting with "nnnn"; "gegegege";"rrrrr";"lllll";"zzzzz";"vvvvv"; ngngngng";"mmmm"

Do you feel vibrations? Is voice easy?

- ❑ RV Messa di voce: start with quietest, pinpoint RV; grow louder evenly over a count of 4, by "opening up," "strengthening sound in your face." Grow quieter evenly over a count of 4: "Hey, yo, hey Joe!"; zebra, voodoo, working, Monday, lit, playing, vigor, rugged, nerve, zodiac, nonsense, metal, log, race

Using a filled-in circle, indicate how your voice is today, overall, compared to when you first started therapy ("X" shows your rating at the start of therapy) (0 = catastrophic; 10 = exquisitely excellent).

	Start of Therapy	Today
10		
9		
8		
7		
6		
5		
4		
3		
2		
1		
0		

Other comments (successes, difficulties, etc.):______________

Discharge Instructions

Date: ____________________

❑ Ongoing home program: ____________________

❑ Management of temporary voice changes due to illness (e.g. colds, etc.) and/or extensive voice use: ____________________

Stretches

It is helpful to begin each training session with stretches. These will not only stretch out the body in preparation for voice training, but will also calm your mind so that you are optimally prepared to learn. Below is a set of stretches that you can use. You clinician may add or change some of them for you. As a rule of thumb, you should sustain each stretch for about 20-30 seconds, unless otherwise indicated. You can stretch to a point of mild discomfort, but not beyond. Throughout all the exercises, inhale slowly and deeply through your nose, and exhale fully through your mouth. You can add some gentle, comfortable voicing in any of the exercises you wish, but voicing is most useful in the latter ones involving the face, mouth, and throat. Dim the lights, play some pleasant music and.....feel the stretch!

1. Open Heart

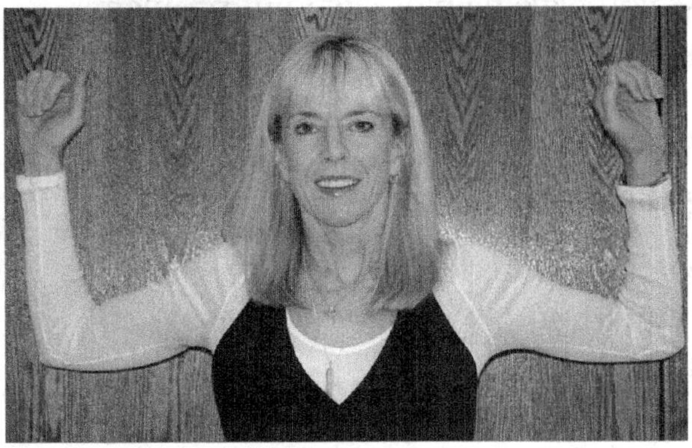

Draw your arms back away from your chest, turning palms forward, and fingers directed upwards. Enjoy the feeling of openness in your chest as you breathe deeply and slowly, inhaling through your nose, exhaling through your mouth.

2. Forward Stretch

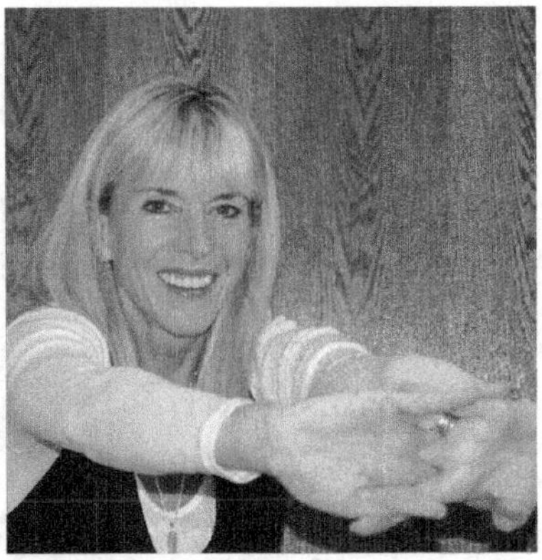

Clasp your hands in front of you, turn them outwards, and gently stretch through your back. Enjoy the feeling of openness in your back as you continue to inhale and exhale as previously).

3. Upper Body Release (Shoulder Shrug)

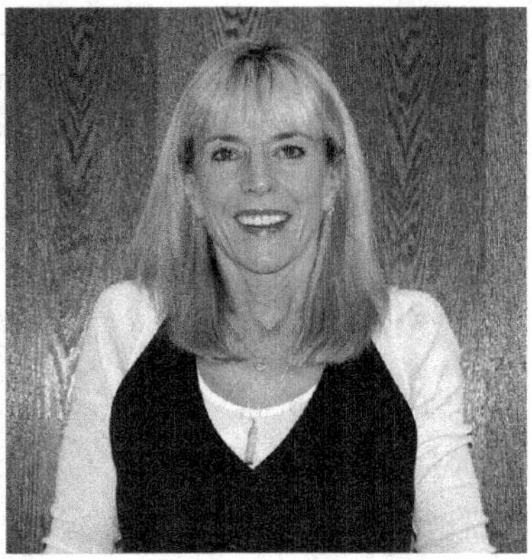

Shrug your shoulders up towards your ears. Then pull your shoulders back and allow them to drop. Repeat 2-3 times. Keep breathing and enjoy!

4. Neck Release

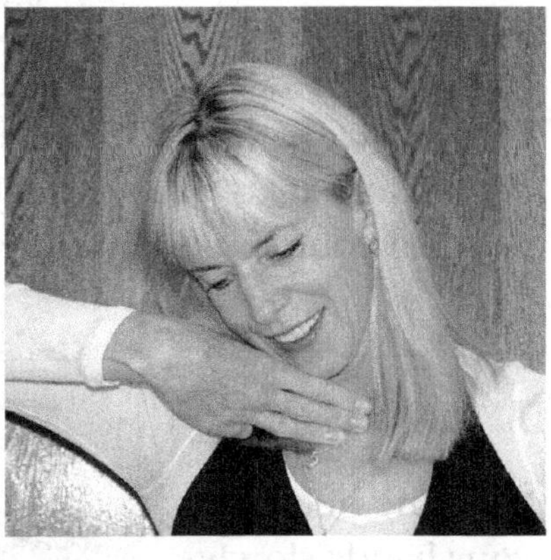

Place three fingers of your right hand under your chin, and tilt your head down to rest on your top finger. Gently sway your head from left to right several times, through a "C-arch," always resting your chin on your fingers. Then when desired, hold in the far right position, feeling the stretch in your left neck. Change hands, by placing three fingers from your left hand under your chin as for the right hand. Hold head in the far left position. End the stretch by swaying your head back and forth through the "C-arch" several times again before removing your fingers from your chin and righting your head.

5. Neck Stretch

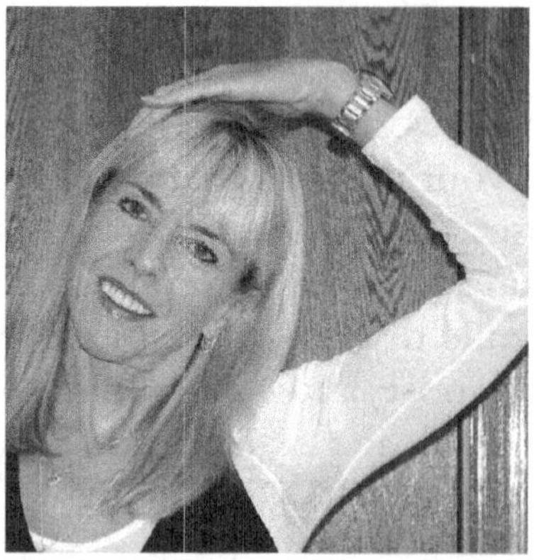

Place your right hand over the top of your head, using your fingers to pull your head gently towards the right. Feel the stretch on the left side of your neck. Hold, extending opposite arm diagonally downwards and pointing fingers. Switch hands and repeat using the left hand, stretching the right side of your neck.

6. Neck Massage

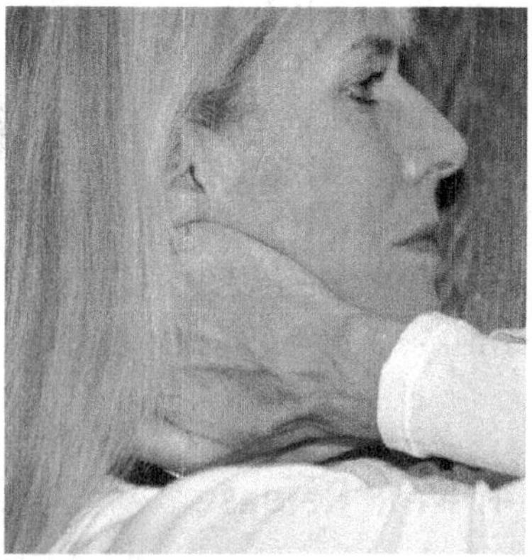

Use the tips of your fingers to press straight into the flesh right under the base of your skull, in the middle. Pull your fingers out towards the sides of the back of your neck. Repeat, as you gradually move down your neck, to your shoulders. Keep breathing!

7. Jaw Massage

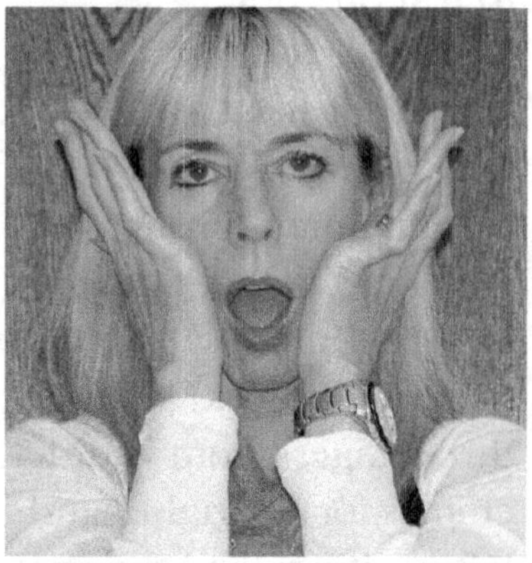

Drag the heels of your hands slowly from your cheek bones down to your lower jaw. You should feel the fleshiness of your jaw muscles under your hands. Feel the muscles release any knots. Repeat several times. Keep breathing; sigh a few gentle "ah"s.

8. Jaw Stretch

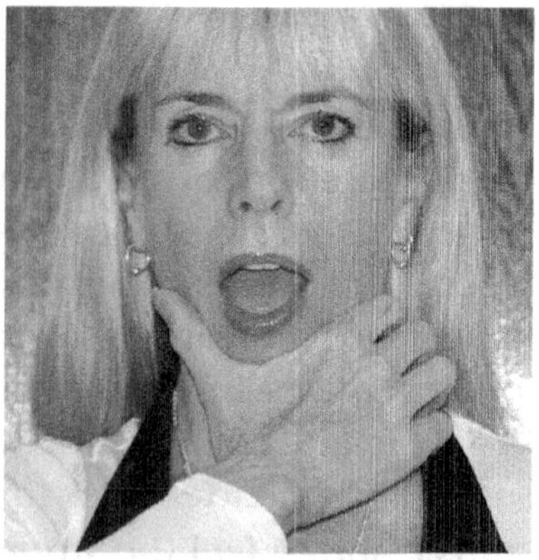

Make a "V" between the thumb and index finger of your preferred hand. Place the "V" over your lower jaw, and pull the jaw gently down and back towards your neck. Extend it through its full range of motion, unless you have pain or jaw joint problems. Breathe gently; sigh on "ah" as you breathe.

9. Lip Release

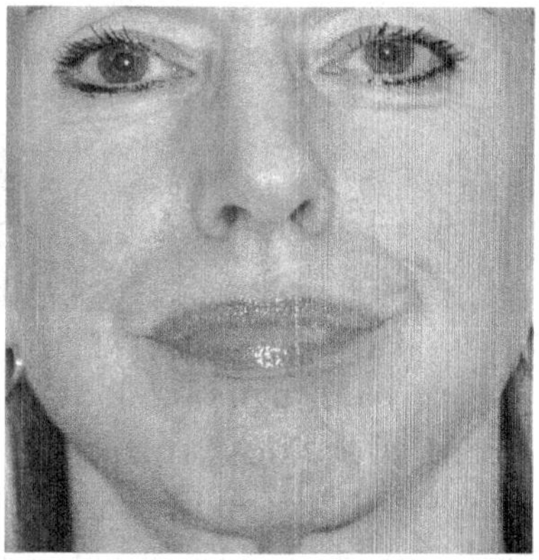

Blow your lips gently apart, so that they vibrate as in a "raspberry." Repeat several times, sighing on a gentle voiced sound. If you have difficulty making "raspberries," you can utter several gentle "puh" sounds, puffing your lips apart as you do so.

10. Tongue Release

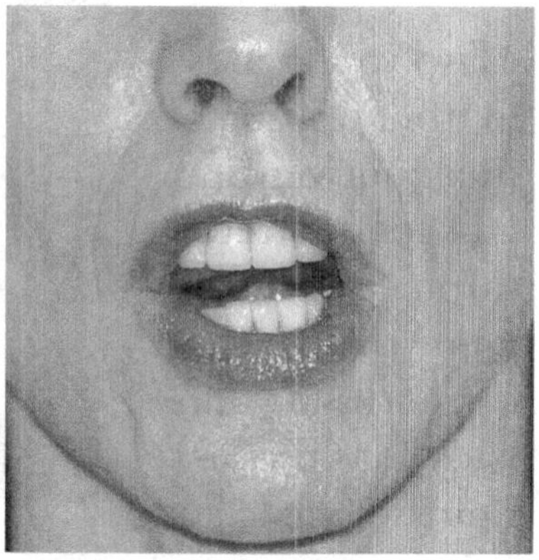

Place your tongue behind your upper teeth, and trill it as for a Spanish "rrrrr." Use gentle voicing as you repeat several trills. If tongue trills are difficult for you, you can produce several sloppy "la la la" sounds to release your tongue.

11. Floor-of-Mouth Release

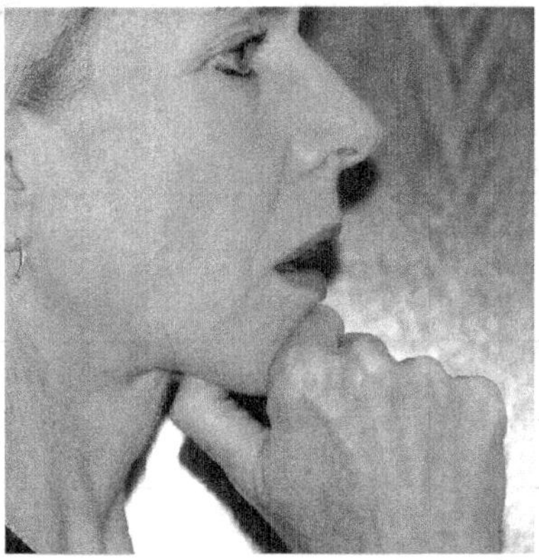

Place your knuckle up under your chin, and massage the "floor of mouth." Let your tongue rest gently on your lower lip as you produce several easy "ah"s.

12. Tongue Stretch

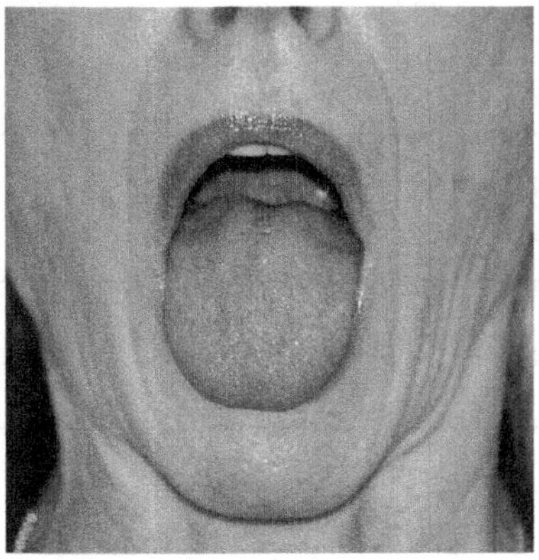

Assume the "lion" posture from yoga by joining your fingers behind you back, raising, your arms behind you as high as you can, and stretch your tongue out of your mouth as far as you can. Breathe; sigh on "ah."

13. Throat Stretch (Yawn)

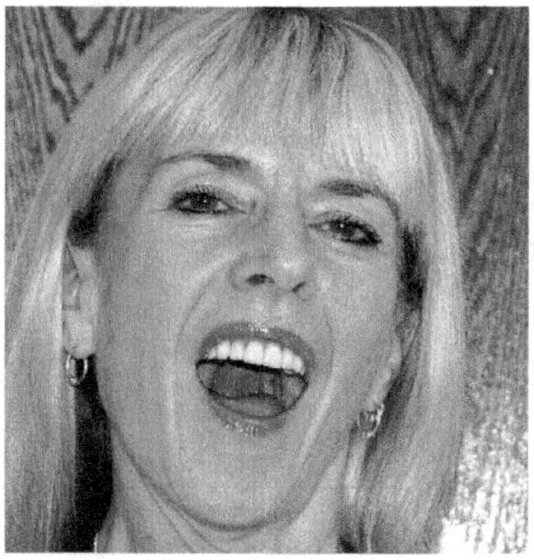

Generate a nice, strong "yawn" as you sigh on "ah." You can combine any of the other exercises you wish with the yawn. For example, you could repeat the Open Heart Stretch, the Upper Body Release (Shoulder Shrug), or the Jaw Massage while yawning and voicing on "ah."

NOTES: